# Sara My Sara

# Sara My Sara

## A Memoir of Friendship and Loss

Florence Wetzel

ISBN: 9798876290809

This book is dedicated to
Victoria and Sarah and Frank

The sorrow bird always has something he can sing about, doesn't he.

Astrid Lindgren<br>*Mio My Mio*, 1954

You can't stop sorrow birds from flying over your head, but you can stop them from building a nest in your hair.

Astrid Lindgren<br>Private letter to Elsa Olenius, 1959

# Contents

# Prologue

## Summer 2020

That hot summer day
I went as always
to Sara's house
in Linden NJ.

As always I walked
Lucky the dog
and as always
I made coffee.

Cup in hand
I went over
to Sara's bed
a hospital bed
in the middle
of the living room.

I laid my hand
on Sara's head.
Before her operation
the previous year
Sara's hair was
long and bronze.
Now it was short
thick and gray
save for a patch
of shiny skin
where her skull
was fused together
by a titanium plate.

Sara crooked her finger
and beckoned me
to come closer.
Her expression
was confused
as it often was
due to the pills
that eased the agony

of the many tumors
growing in her brain.

I took a step forward
and bent down to listen.

'There's a girl over there'
Sara whispered
gesturing nervously
toward the kitchen.
'She told me
she's my daughter.
Is it true?'

I glanced over
at the kitchen.
Sara's daughter
Little Sarah
stood in the corner
tapping on her phone.

A cold finger
touched my heart.

'That's true'
I whispered back.
'The girl is named Sarah.
She's the youngest
of your two daughters
and she loves you
very much.'

Sara nodded
and leaned back.
Her eyes became
a touch calmer.

'OK'
she whispered.
'OK.'

O Sara!
Sara my Sara.

# Part 1

# With Sara

# 2013–18

# Spring 2013 to Spring 2017

It's impossible
to write about Sara
without writing
about my mother.

My mom!
Marion Daisy Wetzel
née Crook
born 1926 in
Coney Island NY.
Another world
in a different time.

Spring 2013
when Sara came
into our lives
my mother was
87 years old
recently widowed
and living in
the small suburb
of Westfield NJ.

My mother was
a suburban diva
reigning over
a four-bedroom house
with a two-car garage
that held a Honda and
her adored Mini Cooper.

My mother also had
a housekeeper
three masseuses
five bank accounts
a Yorkshire terrier
named Lucky
a tuxedo cat
named Mooch
a luxuriant backyard
with a Chinese pavilion
and a pond with ten koi.

Not to mention
eight closets of clothes
and over a thousand
pieces of porcelain.

My mother also had me
her youngest child
recently moved home
at 50 years old.
I had come back
so my mother
wouldn't feel alone
after my father's death.

I had also returned
to help my mother
with practical matters
such as the towering
stacks of documents
and unopened mail
on my father's desk.

My mother's housekeeper
was a Brazilian woman
named Suzana
who for many years
came every Friday
to clean the house.
During the final months
of my father's life
Suzana started coming
three times a week
to help my mother
take care of him.

After my father died
my mother decided
to keep that schedule.
She enjoyed having
Suzana's company
and she liked seeing
the house shiny clean.

Unfortunately
Suzana's mother

suddenly fell ill
and Suzana needed
to return to Brazil
for several months.

That was when Elise
(one of my mother's
three masseuses)
suggested my mother
hire her housekeeper
a woman named Sara
who was also Brazilian.

Great idea!
My mother and Sara
already knew one another
because Sara usually
was working at Elise's
when my mother arrived
for her weekly massage.

The next day Sara came
to my mother's house
with her daughters
Vickie and Little Sarah
who came along
to provide translation.
With their help
my mother and Sara
reached an agreement
on Sara's schedule and pay.

My mother was happy.
Sara was happy.
It was a new phase
in my mother's life.
A widow with
a grown daughter
living at home
and now also Sara
three afternoons a week.

By the way
when Suzana returned
my mother decided

to keep Sara on.
Why have one housekeeper
when you could have two?

I told you she was a diva.

**S**ara.
But her real name
was actually Jussara.

It took a long time
before I found out
Sara's true name.
When I asked why
she used another name
Sara said that Sara
was easier for Americans
to say and remember.

Later I found out
Sara's nickname
was Juju.
What a joyful name!
It fitted her perfectly.

Sara was born
October 17 1962.
I was born
October 14 1962.
We liked to joke
about the fact
that I was older.

She grew up
in Dom Feliciano
in Rio Grande do Sul
in southern Brazil
an area with a large
Polish population
and Sara herself
had Polish roots.

In the late eighties
Sara started writing
letters to Frank
an American man

with Brazilian roots.
They got married
in Brazil in 1991
and afterward Sara
moved to the US.

In 2013 when Sara
started working
for my mother
she and Frank lived
in Linden NJ
with their daughters
Vickie and Sarah
as well as Jordie
a blind poodle
named after
Michael Jordan
who they had saved
from an abusive home.

During her life
Sara had worked
many different jobs
but at that time
she was a housekeeper
for several households
including a man
who had cancer.
Sara evolved into
one of his caregivers
and also helped
empty the house
after his death.

Sara was tall and slim
with long straight hair
in a unique bronze color.
She had big glasses
and high cheekbones.
A broad smile
slightly crooked.

In my mother's house
Sara worked hard
usually wearing

tight white pants
and flowery shirts
often with her phone
clamped between
her shoulder and ear.

Despite her duties
as a housekeeper
I never saw Sara
disheveled or unkempt.
Just like my mother
Sara had mastered
the art of keeping
her glamour intact
in all circumstances.

One of many reasons
Sara fit so smoothly
into my mother's heart.

Sara grew up speaking
Portuguese and Spanish
and began learning English
in her twenties.

I myself learned Swedish
when I was in my fifties
but despite years of study
I was often self-conscious
when I tried to speak.

Sara on the other hand
never hesitated
when speaking English.
She plowed right ahead
confident and talkative
unconcerned with grammar
and other niceties.

Sara's English was unique.
She sometimes added
an extra syllable
for example
saying New York-y
instead of New York.

On the other hand
the last syllable
of many other words
disappeared completely.

I never corrected
Sara's English.
From my experience
with Swedish
I knew it was
more important
to speak freely
than always be right.

Sara had her way
of expressing herself
and slowly I became
used to her English
just as Sara became
used to my English.

There was however
one mystery.
How could my mother
with her failing hearing
and refusal to wear
her expensive hearing aids
understand Sara so well?

No idea.
But I suspect
they had discovered
the language of the heart
a silent understanding
untouched by grammar.


The sorrow bird
had always sung
in my mother's heart.

The best word
to describe my mother
was melancholy.

Not always!
Absolutely not.

My mother liked to laugh
often bursting into song
and peppering her speech
with corny sayings
such as the classic
Don't be mean jelly bean!

My mother enjoyed her life
but in her gaze lurked
a constant undertone
of unprocessed grief.

She lost Robbie
her beloved brother
in a plane crash
August 1 1945
when she was 19.
I doubt she ever
fully recovered
from that loss.

Before she turned 40
my mother had also lost
her mother and father
her cherished Aunt Dotty
and many dogs including
several black poodles
all named Suzy.

My sister Diane
died in 2010
at 50 years old.

My father
died in 2013
after a marriage
of 56 years.

These losses compounded
the previous losses
in an endless chamber
of heartbreak.

My mother was also
a solitary woman.
She and my father were

one of those couples
who lived in a bubble.
My father had
no friends at all.
My mother had
her best friend Elaine
and a few others
most often women
she had employed
in some fashion.

I didn't understand
how much my mother
needed a new friend
until Sara entered
my mother's life
and filled a space
which lo and behold
happened to be shaped
exactly like Sara.

Sara was a joyful bird
with a wide smile
and easy laugh.

She had also had
her share of losses
including her mother
and her father and
one of her sisters.

But unlike my mother
Sara wasn't haunted
by those losses.
The sorrow bird
had never built
a nest in her hair.

Sometimes I thought
my mother and Sara
became so close
because my mother
had lost a daughter
and because Sara
had lost a mother.

Possibly.
But perhaps the reason
was much simpler.

Maybe they
just liked each other.

Maybe they
just clicked.


Sara was empathetic
and radiated warmth
and it didn't take long
until she became
the emotional center
of our household.

Sara was very physical
and liked to hug.
My mother was
not that way
but she wanted
to be that way.

Slowly Sara's
easy physicality
helped my mother
open up.

Our friend Megan
who we met when
my mother hired her
to walk Lucky
once told me
'When I saw Sara
hug your mother
I realized I also
wanted to hug her
so that's when
I started doing it.'

After decades of stiffness
our house was now
alive with hugging.

Sara lived to socialize
and she loved talking
telling stories with
extensive details.

My mother used to
tease her about it
asking jokingly
'Sara are you still talking?'
Whereupon Sara
just laughed.

My mother and Sara
had their own jargon
lots of small things
they liked to repeat
to amuse each other.

Whenever Sara
was about to leave
at the end of the day
she announced cheerfully
'This girl go home!'
which always made
my mother giggle.

Most touching
was that Sara
called my mother
My lady.

Those two words
summed up exactly
how Sara felt
about my mother.

That my mother
was elegant.
That my mother
was part of her.

Of course Sara
was not perfect.

Her biggest flaw
was being late.

Regardless what time
we had agreed upon
Sara always arrived
20 minutes later
sometimes more.

My mother and I were
pathologically punctual.
On the rare occasions
we did come late
we apologized
multiple times
and felt ashamed
the rest of the day.

We discussed Sara's
unique sense of time
and we decided
to just accept it.
It was impossible for us
to be angry at Sara.
We loved her too much.

On the other hand
Sara often stayed late
and my mother
needed to insist
that she go home.
Whereupon Sara
exclaimed brightly
'This girl go home!'

In other words
it worked out.


In the beginning
Sara existed
on the periphery
of my consciousness.

Sara was
my mother's employee
not mine.

Sara was
my mother's confidant
not mine.

We were always
friendly to each other
exchanging a few words
when we crossed paths
in my mother's house
but we never had
a proper conversation.

I also found it
embarrassing
to have someone
clean up after me.
Without my asking
most days my bed
was freshly made
and clean clothes
sat neatly folded
on my desk.

Sara and I coexisted
in my mother's house
physically near
but emotionally far.

Sara worked for my mother
from 2013 to 2017.
During those years
they became close friends.
Best friends even.

My mother and I
also got closer
during that time.
I stopped working as
a freelance proofreader
so I could take care
of my mother and
her complicated life.

I used to joke
that I had become

her personal assistant
although really
it wasn't a joke.

Every morning
my mother drove us
to the Starbucks
in downtown Westfield
in her black-and-yellow
Mini Cooper
which she called
the Bumblebee.

My mother was
the queen of Starbucks.
She knew everyone
and was well-respected
due to her advanced age
and friendly manner.

Everyone enjoyed
my mother's glamour
her long pink nails
dangling earrings
and leopard-print beret
perched on top of
champagne-colored hair.

Each morning
my mother and I
took our places
at her usual table
by the window.

I bought our breakfast
and studied Swedish
while my mother
drank black coffee
and ate a croissant
while reading the paper
and chatting with her pals
especially her favorites
Ricky and Ken.

As soon as my mother's
black coffee cooled off

I stopped studying
and fetched her a refill.
My mother could not bear
lukewarm coffee.

After breakfast
my mother usually went
to a beauty appointment
while I took care
of practical matters.

When I had time
I also took care
of my own life.

I wanted one day
to move to Sweden
and my main activity
was studying Swedish.

I also had a social life
mostly 12-step meetings
coffee with friends
daily yoga classes.

And yes I had
my own problems
including a relationship
that crashed
or rather
never took flight.

But mostly my life
revolved around my mother
and we became closer
than we had ever been
in the previous decades.


There was however
one caveat.

Besides our mornings
at Starbucks and
brief conversations
during the day
I almost never sat

with my mother
to talk to her
or listen to her.

I didn't have
the energy for it.

This was not something
I was proud of then
and I'm certainly not
proud of it now.

But as it turned out
that gap was the place
where Sara entered
my mother's life.
That was the opening
where their friendship
took root and bloomed.

In the afternoons
it was a pleasure
to come home
from doing errands
or studying Swedish
and find the two of them
huddled together.

Sometimes they stood
in the kitchen
chatting and laughing
but mostly they sat
on the flowered sofa
by the wall-length window.

The sofa looked out
on the verdant backyard
a magical place with
roses and daylilies
irises and daffodils
and a half dozen
hanging bird feeders
shaped like houses.

There was even
a Chinese pavilion

and a little pond
with a wooden bridge
where colorful koi
swam round and round.

My mother and Sara
drank tea and talked
intently about their lives
with Lucky the dog
nestled between them.

The warmth of their
blossoming friendship
lit up our house and
their frequent laughter
silenced the sorrow bird
lurking in the corner.

**M**y friendship with Sara
developed slowly.

There wasn't any
exact moment
but the day came
when Sara and I
became a team.
Two people
united in our desire
to keep my mother alive.

The first few years
I lived with my mother
her health was stable.
But slowly she became
weak and brittle.
The woeful song
of the sorrow bird
gradually became
impossible to ignore.

That was when
Sara and I
started to talk
one-on-one

about my mother
and her care.

When my mother saw
Sara and I together
she asked sharply
'Are you two
talking about me?'

Sara and I tried
to look innocent
but yes it was true.

If Sara and I were talking
we were most likely
talking about my mother.

We talked about
my mother's declining eyesight
and her refusal to stop
driving her Mini Cooper
despite several small collisions
which my mother would
never call accidents.

We talked about
my mother's declining hearing
and her reluctance to wear
her expensive hearing aids
except when dining out
where she usually
removed them and
left them behind
beside her plate.

We talked about
my mother's wobbly balance
and her refusal to
install handrails
by the staircase or
in the bathrooms.
My mother proclaimed
'I don't want it to look
like an old person
lives in my house!'

She was 89
when she said that.

We talked about
my mother's arthritis
which made it impossible
for her to do simple things
like open a bottle of pills
or tie her own shoelaces.

We talked about
my mother's bad habit
of writing large checks
to anyone who asked
which further shrank
her shrinking bank account.

We talked about the fact
that my mother was now
a danger to herself and others.
To all of Westfield actually
when one considered
how recklessly she drove
her posh Bumblebee.

We also talked about
Sara's schedule and salary
which I had become
responsible for
just as I had become
responsible for
everything else
in my mother's life.

Those were the things
Sara and I talked about.
Every conversation wove
a tapestry of friendship
that only got stronger
as my mother got weaker.

During those last years
with my mother
I was scared.

I had been a daughter
for over 50 years
and now my mother
was weaker than me.

She used to be
responsible for me
but now I was
responsible for her.

I didn't want that.
I wanted the mother
I always had.

A self-sufficient woman
who traveled the world
(Asia Africa Antarctica
dozens of countries
too many to name).

An independent woman
who took care of
her own life
by herself.

A caring woman
who took care of me
when I needed help.

That woman
was fading away.
Slowly at first
then faster and faster.
Like running downhill
gaining momentum as
you hurtle toward the end.

Sometimes
I looked around for
the responsible adult
who would take care of
this new world
I found myself in.

But the only one
I ever saw
was me.

No that wasn't
entirely true.
When I looked around
I also saw Sara.

What a relief!
I wasn't all alone
after all.

Thanks Sara.


The thing my mother
hated the most
was that our roles
had become reversed.

One time in Starbucks
my mother couldn't
button her jacket
due to the crippling
arthritis in her hands.
I had to kneel and
button it for her
just as she had
buttoned my coat
many decades before.

My mother didn't like
me being the boss.
Often when I made
a simple request
she answered me
highly sarcastic
'Yes mom!'

Other times my mother
said accusingly
'You're bossy!'
Whereupon I answered
also accusingly
'You're stubborn!'

My mother's resistance
was understandable.
As her body faded
her willfulness was

the only thing
she had left.

But at the same time
her willfulness made
my life difficult.

Often I told my mother
that she was being sassy.
Which was merely
a kinder way to say
childish
illogical
stubborn
hard to handle
self-sabotaging.

It wasn't easy
taking care of someone
who didn't want
to be taken care of.

### Sara
on the other hand
had a magic effect
on my mother
that surely saved
my mother's life
countless times
those last years.

For example
when I suggested
moving the microwave
from a high shelf
down to the counter
so my mother would
avoid dropping
piping-hot food
on her own head
my mother answered
strong and determined
'No.'

But as soon as Sara
asked my mother
the very same thing
my mother replied
compliant and obedient
'Sure!'

Clearly it was easier
for my mother
to accept help
from Sara
rather than
her own daughter.

I never took it personally.
I was just thankful
my mother listened
to anyone at all.

What mattered
was the result
namely keeping
my mother safe
something she could
no longer manage
by herself.

Naturally it's risky
when an elderly woman
who is wealthy and
let's face it
a touch eccentric
becomes fond of
listens to and obeys
only one other person.

I didn't think of that
then
but I certainly realize it
now.

My mother
would have done
anything for Sara.
She would have

given Sara money
or bought her
expensive things
if Sara had asked.

But Sara never
asked for anything
and I don't believe
she would have accepted
if my mother had offered.
Which maybe my mother did
without me knowing.

Sara was an honorable woman
who acted from the heart.
I trusted her completely
and that trust
was never exploited.


Everything changed
June 2016
after my mother
had a heart procedure.

The operation was intended
to make my mother stronger
but unfortunately
it made her weaker
and after that
she was never the same.

The procedure went well
and my mother was
about to be discharged.
But one morning when
I arrived at the hospital
her green eyes were wild
and her pale mouth
tight and shaky.

My mother but
at the same time
not my mother.

The sorrow bird
sat behind her eyes
and screamed.

Turns out my mother
had an infection.
It took 13 days
until the infection
finally disappeared
and during that time
my mother lost
her physical strength.

Sara was beside me
the whole time.
She took care of
our home and pets
and sat by my mother
at the hospital
whenever I needed
to take a break.

Finally my mother
returned home.
Now she was a weak
90-year-old woman
with a frail heart
and iron will.

It was probably then
Sara and I became
friends for real.

We both understood
what was at stake
and we formed a team
with a common goal
of keeping my mother
alive and safe
happy if possible
and always with
her glamour intact.

My mother became
weaker and weaker

and at the same time
harder to handle.

Fear became my
constant companion
as was the sorrow bird
hovering above me
and drawing nearer
with each passing day.

I dealt with my fear
via yoga classes
12-step meetings
studying Swedish
coffee with friends.

The best medicine
was always Sara.
The minute her blue jeep
swung into the driveway
my heart beat slower.

'Mom!' I called out.
'Sara's here!'

My mother's eyes
lit up with joy.

Lucky barked
and ran to the door
to welcome his friend.

Everything
came into balance
as soon as Sara
stepped inside.

As if the whole house
could finally exhale.


The biggest conflict
I had with my mother
concerned her driving.

Her sight had gotten worse
which affected every aspect
of her life and mine.

One day she said
'Everything has
become so dark.'

Whenever my mother
drove us to Starbucks
it was terrifying to see
her difficulty staying
on her side of the road
and how she fumbled
after the handbrake
blind and unsure.

'Mom' I begged her.
'It's time to stop driving.
You don't see well enough.'

'I can see far!'
she answered.

'But you also need
to see at close range.
You're going to crash
or run someone over.'

'I have insurance!'
she replied.

'Mom! That is
not the point.'

After the heart procedure
my mother's doctor
forbade her to drive
for six whole weeks.
Such a relief!

Not long afterward
when I was about
to travel to Sweden
Sara said to me
'Hide the car keys
to both the cars
including the spare keys.
Don't let me know
where you put them
so I won't have to

lie to your mother
when she asks me
for the keys.'

That's what I did
thank goodness
because the first time
I went to drive
after my return
I found my mother's
colorful keyring
lying in the front seat
of the Honda.

Presumably she had
left the keyring there
after getting into the car
despite the doctor's ban.
That was when
she discovered
the ignition key
was missing
from the ring.

Sara told me
my mother had torn
through the house
like a hurricane
on several occasions
determined to find
her missing car keys.

Luckily she never
found my hiding spot
which was underneath
my sock-drawer liner.

At my mother's next
doctor's appointment
I mentioned our
driving problem.
Which was when
the doctor forbade
my mother to drive.
Forever.

Immediately my mother
declared her intention
to get an independent test
in order to prove
she was fit to drive.

The doctor looked at me.
'Don't worry' he said.
'She won't pass.'

I never gave the keys
back to my mother.
Gradually she stopped
searching for them.

However
from then on
whenever we met
somebody new
my mother always
introduced me
by saying:

'This is Florence
my youngest daughter.
She's the one
who took away
my car keys.'

I told you she was sassy.

**M**y mother's greatest worry
was who would take
Lucky and Mooch
after she died.

It's impossible to write
about my mother and Sara
without mentioning Lucky.

Lucky!
A big Yorkshire terrier
with a silky gold coat.
A dog no one wanted
who had been rejected
from three different homes

until he landed
at my mother's house
March 2012.

I know the exact date
because my mother
had a Post-it note
above my father's desk
LUCKY CAME TO ME
MARCH 8 2012.

Lucky was not
an easy dog.
He was nervous
and barked
long and loud
for no reason at all.
But he had a heart
as big as a house
and he was always
fiercely protective
of my mother.

The first evening
I moved in with her
Lucky jumped on my bed
and growled savagely
his furry face twisted
into an angry scowl.

'Lucky!' I exclaimed.
'What's going on?'

He stopped at once
and licked my hand.
Which is when
I understood
Lucky was just
letting me know
who was the boss.

When Sara started
working in our house
Lucky never once
challenged her.
Just like my mother

he was happy with
Sara being the boss.

Lucky and Sara
loved each other.
When she pulled
into the driveway
Lucky ran at once
to the garage door
wagging his tiny tail.

When Sara came in
she lifted up Lucky
and held his face to hers
in a nose-to-nose kiss
which made Lucky's eyes
sparkle with euphoria.

I loved Lucky
with all my heart.
I saw him as
my dog-brother.

I walked him
several times each day
which added up to
thousands of walks
during the four years
I lived with my mother.

Lucky slept alternately
with my mother and me.
The first part of the night
he stayed with her
then in the wee hours
he left her room and
padded down the hallway
to join me in my room.

Despite my love for Lucky
I knew I couldn't take him
after my mother's death
because I planned
to move to Sweden.
My mother needed
someone willing

to adopt her loyal
and difficult dog.

One day I came home
and found my mother
and Sara and Lucky
sitting on the sofa
their eyes shining.

My mother told me
that she and Sara
had made a pact.
In the event
one of them died
the survivor would
adopt the other's
treasured dog.

Sara of course
lived with her family
so from her side
the agreement was
mostly symbolic.
But still that promise
meant the world
to both of them and
during her last year
my mother often
mentioned their pact.

As my mother used to say
'Love me
love my dog.'

**A**fter her heart procedure
my mother decided
to use her insurance and
hire a full-time health aide.

Not that my mother
needed constant help.
Not yet anyway.
But the more often
someone was around

to keep an eye on her
the better for everyone.

My mother also wanted
to make it easier for me
to travel to Sweden.
By that time I went on
fewer and fewer trips
which had become
shorter and shorter.

A full-time aide
was a good idea
except for one
important detail.

I asked my mother
'If someone starts
working full-time
what about Sara?'

My mother stared at me
as if I was crazy.
'Of course Sara is staying!'

That was my mother.
Why have one
when you can have two?

The new woman started
just before I left
on a four-week trip
to Sweden.

I flew away
secure and happy
because my mother was
secure and happy.

I called home daily
and on the third day
Sara informed me
my mother had fired
the new woman.

Why?
No particular reason.
Just because.

Sara was scheduled
to work her usual
four days a week
but she promised
to come daily
until I returned.

Two months later
I took a 12-day cruise
on the coast of Norway
to research my book
The Woman Who Went Overboard.

The cruise was a present
from my mother
to say thank you
for helping her.

(Thanks Mom.)

Before I left
my mother hired
another woman
full-time.

The ship's internet
was unreliable
so a few days passed
before I got in touch.

Which is when
Sara told me
my mother had fired
this woman as well.

Why?
No particular reason.
Just because.

Exactly as before
Sara promised
to come daily
until I returned.

I logged out of Skype
and closed my laptop
on the wooden desk
in my little cabin.

My elderly mother was
thousands of miles away
but her strong will
still reached me
in the middle of
a black and icy sea
in a ship traveling north
toward the Arctic Circle.

I told you she was stubborn.


When I returned home
my mother and I sat
at the kitchen island
for a serious talk
about her habit
of firing people
she had just hired.

My mother told me
she didn't want
any of those women
inside her house.

There was no point
reminding my mother
that she was the one
who had hired them.
Instead I asked
'What *do* you want?'

My mother was 90
painfully thin
shaky and brittle
with impaired vision
and minimal hearing.
Nonetheless
she banged her fist
on the kitchen island

and declared vehemently
'I want Sara!'

All right then.

January 2017
I gave Sara a letter
to bring home and
read with her family
asking if she could
leave her other jobs
and work for us full-time.

I explained that
I didn't know how long
the job would last
because I didn't know
how much longer
my mother would live.
But if Sara wanted
she could stay on
after my mother's death
to help empty the house
and then receive
severance pay.

Sara said yes at once.

Our relief was enormous.
We couldn't use
my mother's insurance
to pay Sara's salary
because Sara was not
an accredited caregiver.
But even if it took
my mother's last penny
Sara was worth it.

And so Sara started coming
all day every day
to everyone's benefit.

That period
was also hard
for my mother.

Sometimes she said
in a distant little voice
'I don't understand
why I'm still here.'

My mother didn't mean
here in Westfield.
She meant being alive
altogether.

The first time
she said that
I donned my most
animated voice
and eagerly recited
all the reasons why
we needed her.

But over time
I let my mother
say those words
without trying
to change them
into something more
comfortable for me.

That was her truth
and I had to let her
say it in peace.

It was not my task
to silence the sorrow bird
no matter how much
that particular song
grated my heart.


Spring 2017.
The final months
of my mother's life.

The days were filled
with multicolored pills
endless doctor visits
several hospital stays.

Westfield was alive
with blossoming trees
and dazzling flowers
but for us it was
a cheerless time
a helpless time
as my mother
ebbed away.

Sara was beside
my mother and me
every single day
except Sundays.

The less my mother
said yes to me
the more my mother
said yes to Sara.
'I want Sara!'

We tried to create
a good life for
my vanishing mother.

On the days when
she was strong enough
to leave the house
I dressed my mother
and took her to Starbucks
for a cup of black coffee.

Sara joined us there and
spent the rest of the day
with my mother
taking her to various
beauty appointments.

Her beloved hairdresser
John at Salon Visage
every Friday morning.
Facials with Barbara
every two weeks.
Weekly manicures
biweekly pedicures.
A shot of Botox
every third month

including an injection
six weeks before she died.

I told you she was a diva.

But now a fragile one
who needed someone
to keep an eye on her
while she showered
and also required
an arm to clutch
as she teetered
across the street and
up and down stairs.

It felt as if my mother
was always in danger.
Although surely
the greatest threat
to my mother was
my mother herself
and her stubborn denial
that she was old
and needed help.

Sometimes
her obstinacy
was admirable.
Now and then
it was amusing.
But most often
it was trying
exhausting
frightening
and it made me
extremely sad.


In those final months
Sara truly became
part of our family.

A quirky clan
composed of
a fading matriarch
an adult daughter

a nervous dog
a snooty cat
a pond full of koi
and now also Sara.

A resilient tribe
full of love and
able to withstand
the occasional conflict
and the ominous presence
of a circling sorrow bird.

Later Little Sarah
told me she often
said to her mother
'You seem like you
actually look forward
to going to work!'

We all looked forward
to Sara coming to work.
Everyone waited for
the moment when Sara
walked into the house
and completed our family.

That's how it was
all day every day
to everyone's benefit.


During my mother's
final illness
she was once again
in the hospital.

Even though my mother
was gray and weak
we still had hope.

And why not?
According to the wise
Portuguese proverb:
Hope is the last to die.

One late afternoon
I was in an Uber

going home after
a long hospital day
with my mother
when I got a call from
an unknown doctor.

My mother needed
an emergency operation
and it was possible
she would not survive.

Of course I called Sara.
She was off that day
to go to Vickie's
college graduation
and a party afterward.

But never mind all that!
Sara was on her way.

At the hospital
my mother was
back in her room
after the operation.
She was sedated and
lying completely still
with closed eyes.

Gradually we became
six women around
my mother's bed.
Sara was there
with her daughters
all of them wearing
pretty party dresses.
The girls sat in chairs
beside my mother's bed
stroked her arms and
whispered to her softly.

After almost an hour
to everyone's surprise
my mother woke up.
She was alive!

My mother was so feeble
she was almost transparent.
But when we explained
about the operation
my mother understood
everything we said.
She was alive!

We talked with her
a little bit more
then she fell
into a deep sleep.

The next day
my mother was frail
but conscious.

Her dear friend Annemarie
one of her three masseuses
visited that afternoon.
They drank black coffee
shared a brownie
chatted and laughed.

As it turned out
that was the last time
my mother ate solid food.

Not long afterward
she sank into
an unshakable sleep.
Not comatose
but completely still
with eyes closed
as she hovered
beyond our reach.

Two days later
during the quiet hours
of early morning rounds
her handsome doctor
informed me that
my mother was not
going to get better.

Yes there were
a few things
he could try
but regardless of
anything he did
my mother had
at best
two weeks left.

That meant
two more weeks
of doctors and nurses
poking and prodding
her fading body.

Two more weeks
of suffering
on top of the recent
weeks of suffering
which were intolerable
both for my mother
and those who loved her.

This was the endgame
just a few pieces
on the chessboard
with no way left
to save the king
or in this case
the queen.

'Alternatively'
the handsome doctor said
'we can stop all the medicine
and when the pain comes
give your mother morphine.'

'If we do that'
I stammered
'how many days
would she have left?'

He looked me
straight in the eye.
'She won't last the week.'

It was Monday.
Which gave
my mother
five days
at most.

And so it was.
The medicine ceased and
a nurse hung a picture
on my mother's door
of a lit white candle
on a black background.

A discreet way
of informing everyone
that the end was now.

**M**y mother
remained unreachable
the rest of the day.

I was certain
she would never
wake up again.

O mom!
Were you really
already gone?

No more black coffee
hot and never lukewarm?

No more long pink nails
Botox treatments
leopard-print beret
teetering on top of
champagne-colored hair?

No more sassy comments
mischievous smiles
spontaneous songs
corny sayings like
Don't be mean jelly bean?

If I didn't have
so very much
to take care of

my heart would have
imploded from grief.

But guess what!
The next morning
when I stepped into
my mother's room
I found her
sitting up in bed
eyes open wide
completely awake.

'Hello' she said.

I was dumbstruck.
'Hey Mom!'

The handsome doctor
entered the room.
He said he had
seen this happen
many times before.
Take away the drugs
and the patient
comes back to life.

What he didn't say
but what I knew
was that the endgame
could not be reversed.
The queen remained
teetering on the brink
still dying with
less than a week
left on earth.

My mother looked at
her handsome doctor
and said loudly
'I want a glass of wine.'

He laughed.
'Unfortunately we can't
give you that here.
Wait until you're home.'

My mother raised an eyebrow.
That was not the answer
she had been hoping for.

**I** called Sara at once.

It was seven in the morning
and she was scheduled
to relieve me at noon.

'My mom's awake!'
I exclaimed.
'Come now!'

Sara was not late that day.
When she ran into
the hospital room
a half hour later
my mother joked
'I thought I had fired you.'

Sara smiled widely.
'You can't get rid of me
that easily.'

I stepped out of the room
and left them alone
so they could enjoy
each other's company
as they always did.

Leaving my mother
with Sara
felt the same as
leaving my mother
with myself.

**S**ure enough
the pain came.
It roared through
my mother's body
and decimated her.

My mother
started receiving
intravenous morphine.

Which is when
the doctor told me
it was time to create
a home hospice
so my mother
could die there.

My first thought was
'Absolutely not!'
I wasn't a nurse
and the thought that
my immense ignorance
might hurt my mother
scared me senseless.

I didn't express this
to the doctor.
Instead I listened
while he explained
how the changeover
would take place.

He introduced me to
a home hospice lady
whose job it was
to transfer my mother
from the hospital
to our house.

While the woman talked
I listened and nodded
fear blazing through
each cell of my body.

I also talked with
a nurse named Dean
a friendly young man
in his late twenties.

I wanted to shout
'You're all asking
too much from me!
Why can't my mother
stay in the hospital
with people who know

how to take care of
someone who's dying?'

Instead I said
tentatively
'Isn't it better
for my mother
to stay here and
get professional help?'

Dean answered
'Even though
she's on morphine
your mother will know
she's at home.
Home is home.'

That was the moment
when I changed my mind.
My mother loved her home.
Everyone knew that.

Besides which
there was something
my mother told me
numerous times.

'When I'm like this'
(she closed her eyes
turned her head and
opened her mouth
wide like a fish)
'please put me
next to the window
looking out over
my backyard.'

I promised my mother
that it would be so.
Now it was time
to keep that promise.

Home is home.
Dean's words
became a mantra
that comforted me

and gave me the strength
to do what I absolutely
did not want to do.

Thanks Dean.

It took time to
sort out the details.

Booking the ambulance.
Arranging hospital staff
to take my mother
down to the ambulance.
Timing the morphine
so my mother wouldn't
wake up in the middle
of her last journey
in terrible agony.

We also needed
to prepare everything
at home in Westfield.
Home health aides
a hospital bed
morphine.

Sara was with me
every step of the way.
I was at the hospital
and she was at home
getting things ready.
We called each other
throughout the day
updating one another
on our positions.
Like conducting
a military operation
but with cell phones
instead of walkie-talkies.

During the ambulance ride
my mother moaned
at every single bump
despite the morphine
she had just received.

I was terrified
and bewildered
and I held her hand
while the sorrow bird
hunched in a corner
and whimpered.

**M**y mother's house
became a hospice.
Now I was the one
responsible for her.

On the surface
I was composed
but underneath
I was trembling.

Not just because
I was on the verge
of losing my mother
(mom!)
but because my mother
was once again
my responsibility
and she was
so very sick
so very dying.

We would have help
from home health aides
round the clock.
I was grateful for that
until I found out
it was illegal for them
to administer morphine.
You could ask
if they were willing
but it was risky
since they weren't trained.

The home hospice lady
told me this and
my placid surface
cracked open.

It was one thing
to organize
my mother's pills
in a plastic box.
But now I needed
to give her morphine
or instead rely on
untrained strangers.

The only person
who I could trust
with something
this important
was Sara.

I asked her
if she was willing
to help me give
my mother morphine.

Sara said yes
at once.

Of course she did.

The hospice lady
taught us how
to carefully draw
the liquid morphine
into a syringe.

She showed us how
to insert the syringe
all the way back
in my mother's mouth
so the precious liquid
would not trickle out.

She demonstrated how
to press the plunger
and then gently
pull out the syringe.

Sara and I watched
with greatest attention.
This had to be done
exactly right

or my mother's
unbearable pain
would once again
engulf her.

At the hospital
a doctor told me
my mother's cells
were now exploding.
That was certainly
something I wanted
to spare her from.

And so during
my mother's last
hours on earth
(36 to be exact)
both Sara and I
kept her suffering
at a merciful distance.
We helped her sink
deeper and deeper
into a place I hoped
was free of torment
and silent as nirvana.

We carried out
my mother's wishes
exactly as she wanted.

She lay with
her eyes closed
head to the side
and mouth open
wide like a fish
next to the window
looking out over
her cherished backyard.

Those final days
were sunny and mild
and those final nights
cool and still.

In the magical backyard
birds fluttered beside
colorful wooden houses.
The flowers radiated
springtime perfume
and the brilliant koi
swam round and round.

My mother's gardener Bill
who she loved like a son
worked in the yard
those final days.
The underlying hum
of landscape work
and Bill's conversation
with his employees
drifted in and out
of our sad house
all day long.

One disappointment
was Lucky and Mooch
who refused to lie
next to my mother
on the hospital bed.

The first time
I lifted Lucky
onto the bed
he went up to
my mother's face
and smelt her lips.
He drew his head
back in distaste and
hopped off the bed.

I tried with Mooch
but he also declined
to stay on the bed.

They did however
sit on the sofa
where they watched
my mother and

the many people
coming to her bedside.

They never let my mother
out of their sight
but they refused
to lie next to her
like they always did.

A mystery.
It was unfortunate and
not what I wanted
but I had to respect
their decision.

The hours passed
in a misty dream.

At night
I set the alarm
every two hours
so I could give
my mother morphine.

In the dark silence
I filled the syringe
and inserted it gently
into her mouth.
I pushed the plunger
and fed her oblivion.

Sara was there
all day every day
as was a changing rota
of home health aides.

Numerous friends
came to say goodbye
including my mother's
best friend Elaine.

Elaine!
The same age
as my mother
a thin stylish woman
of impeccable taste

whose purse and shoes
always matched her
flawlessly tailored clothes.
No one gave better gifts
than Elaine.

My mother had met Elaine
thanks to their shih tzus
Elaine's dog Henry
the smelliest shih tzu
in the entire world
and my mother's dog Cookie
who was Lucky's predecessor.

My mother and Elaine
shared a mutual love
of fine dining and
they often ate out
at their favorite
local restaurant
Rosie's Wine Bar.

When Elaine visited
our home hospice
she stood by the bed
stroked my mother's hair
and spoke with her
in a hushed voice.

I left them in peace
but one moment
as I walked past
I heard Elaine
whisper tenderly
'Goodbye my beautiful friend.'


**M**y mother lay
in the hospital bed
and didn't react
to anything at all.

Her eyes remained
tightly closed.
Not a single sound
escaped her mouth.

Sara and I had
a final conversation
with my mother
as she floated atop
soft waves of morphine.

We told her
'You can go now!
Don't worry about
Lucky and Mooch.
And don't worry
about us either.
Go!'

I'm sure Sara also
had private last words
with my mother when
I wasn't in the room.

Later that afternoon
after everyone had left
apart from an aide
I sat on the bed and
took my mother's hand.

I said to her
in a sad little voice
'I love you mom.'

I almost fell
off the bed
when my mother
pressed my hand.
With her eyes
still firmly shut
she curved her lips
into an elegant smile.

Aha!
Was it possible
she had been aware
the entire time?

That was my mother.
Always full of surprises.

I told you she was sassy.

**M**y mother died
during her second night
in home hospice.

Just after midnight
I went to her bed
with a full syringe
of morphine.

In the dark silence
I carefully placed
the plastic syringe
into her mouth
and released
the magic liquid.

That's when I noticed
my mother's face
was stiff.

That's when I realized
my mother was dead.

Time split
into two parts.

A silent fracture
with my mother
on one side
and me
on the other.


**A** nurse came
to the house
and confirmed
my mother's death.

The nurse and the aide
gave their condolences
and then went home.

I remained alone
with my mother
as I waited for
the funeral home

to come and
take her away.

The room was dark
save for the tiny
white Christmas lights
that glittered at night
in the enchanted backyard.

I set up a diffuser
with lavender oil
and played the CD
of mellow Asian flutes
my mother always put on
before she went to sleep.

Mute and exhausted
I took a seat beside
my mother's bed.

The sorrow bird
hovered above my head
and wept into the air.

That was the moment
when Lucky and Mooch
after having watched
from a distance
for two whole days
jumped up on the bed.

Lucky snuggled into
my mother's hip and
Mooch lay his chin
on my mother's thigh.

They stayed like that
until the doorbell rang
and two sturdy men
from the funeral home
entered the house.

'Don't worry'
one of them said.
'We're going to take
very good care of her.'

That night
I barely slept.

I woke early
painfully aware
that it was time
to start shouldering
the crushing tsunami
of responsibility
I had just inherited.

But first
I needed to dispose of
my mother's medicine.
Particularly the morphine.

For someone like me
with a history of addiction
the bottles of morphine
sitting in the refrigerator
vibrated with danger.

My sorrow was bottomless
and I longed for oblivion
while one of mankind's
most potent painkillers
lurked nearby and
murmured darkly.

At eight o'clock
I left the house.
A quiet Saturday
in late May with
a clear blue sky
and mild breeze.

Wearing a flowered dress
I hopped on my pretty
mint-green bike
a birthday present
from my mother
some years before.

I rode slowly along
the wide avenues of
the charming suburb

past stately Victorian homes
their front yards blazing
with colorful flowers
and blossoming trees.

In the white basket
attached to the front
of my green bicycle
I had a bag of pills and
two bottles of morphine.

First I rode to
the police station.
In the lobby stood
an old mailbox
for dropping off
leftover pills.

Then I rode to
the only pharmacy
willing to take back
liquid medicine.

When the clerk
opened at 8:30
she found me
outside the door.
What a relief
to finally give over
those two bottles!

I cycled home
under the open sky
and that's when I began
the first day of my life
without my mother.


What am I supposed to do
without you?

How am I supposed to go on
without you?

How am I supposed to live
on this earth
without you?

Sara came.

Even though
it was Saturday.
Even though
my mother was
no longer there
to take care of.

Sara stayed with me
the whole day.
We spoke quietly
as we removed
every trace of
the home hospice.

The only thing left
was the hospital bed
scheduled for removal
the coming Monday.

We made the bed with
a clean white sheet
and lay a red rose
on the emptiness.

The delicate song
of the sorrow bird
floated through the room
on a breeze soft and sad.

Mom!
Where was my mother?

My mother was
invisible yet present
like a gentle mist
a drifting scent
a passing shadow.
She was everywhere
but at the same time
she was nowhere.

A woman had lived
a long and full life
from 1926 to 2017
and now she was gone.

# Summer 2017

After my mother died
a new phase started
for Sara and me.

My plan was to go to
Sweden in September.
That gave us three months
to empty the house
and prepare it for sale.

Previously Sara had
spent most of her day
with my mother.
Now there was
only Sara and I
and most of her day
would be spent with me.

The sorrow bird was
also there of course.
Its specter perched
in all the corners
of our grieving home.

Each morning
when I awoke
that bleak summer
I felt suffocated
by the day ahead.

Emptying and revamping
a four-bedroom house
where a family had lived
almost five decades
was a thankless job
and I was the epicenter
of the endless activity
required to make it salable.

A particular slice of hell
was the oil tank
buried in the front yard.
The tank had been

leaking oil for years
and now it needed
to be removed
and afterward
the polluted soil
had to be replaced.

It was always a comfort
when Sara's blue jeep
drove up the driveway.
She arrived late
of course
but that was OK.

We started our day
at the kitchen island
nursing cups of coffee
with Lucky sitting
snugly on Sara's lap.

We talked through
the day's schedule and
everyone who was due
to come to the house.

Sara was easy to be with
and we worked together
in a serene flow.

The immense loss
we faced every day
wove us closer
building trust
solidarity
sisterhood.

Mom!
Where was my mother?

The house felt like
a railway station.

In came friends
and friends' friends.
Anyone interested
in taking away

furniture books clothes
plants porcelain paintings
was warmly welcome
day and night.

In came our friend and neighbor
Patty the real estate agent.
In came our friend
Patti the lawyer.

In came Bill the landscaper
and his gang of workers.
In came handyman Bill
and his many assistants.

In came Scott the electrician
who my mother also
loved like a son.

In came Cheryl
to write up long lists
of books and jazz records.

In came the exterminator and
the water-sprinkler company.
In came people to fix
the furnace
the chimney
the fireplace
the water softener
and take down
a dead tree.

In came a fleet of companies
to remove the oil tank
and the polluted soil
which meant digging a hole
as big as a Volkswagen
and uprooting my mother's
favorite cherry tree.

In came the home stylist
the antique appraiser
and also Merilyn
with her color wheel
to help me choose

the perfect shade of gray
to paint the walls.

In came the lady
who cleaned the pond
to take the koi.
She ran to her truck
with the fish flopping
in her hands.

In came a company
called 1-800-I Got Junk
who took everything
no one else wanted.

In came Tony D
who bought the last
pieces of furniture
and told me that
if he had a backyard
as private and enclosed
as my mother's
he'd take off his clothes
and walk around naked
all day long.

**D**uring those weeks
I was also at the start
of my mourning.

I kept a tenuous
emotional balance
through yoga classes
12-step meetings
coffee with friends.

I also got strength
from the knowledge
I was taking care of
my mother's treasured
house and garden
and wrapping up
her final business
on this earth.

Sara was the strength
that centered my world.
She helped me survive
the sad hectic months
of that burning-hot summer.

But it wasn't easy.
My sorrow manifested
not only in tears
but also anger
fear
inertia
apathy
overeating.

The worst was the rage
which could erupt
at any moment.

I never got angry at Sara
but the rest of the world
wasn't safe in my company.

Once at a 12-step meeting
a friend said something
innocuous to me
and I snapped at her
for no reason at all.

She looked at me
eyes full of shock
and said quietly
'I have never ever
seen you like this.'

That's when I realized
I was scaring people.
Which scared me.

I had to rein myself in
if I could
and unfortunately
I couldn't always.

One thing
I didn't anticipate

was that I now stood
in my mother's place.

I was a placeholder
the nearest anyone
could come to my mother
now that she was gone.

The house also felt
like a placeholder
for my mother.
Sara and I enjoyed
the cool breeze
of my mother's spirit
that floated silently
in the vacant house.

Likewise my mother's friends
became placeholders for me.
Particularly Maryellen
who worked downtown
at Salon Visage.
A few times a week
I went to the salon
just before it opened
and chatted with her.
I was a lost little bird
whom she gently fed
fresh brewed coffee
and tiny butter cookies.
She listened to me and
she mourned with me.

Thanks Maryellen.


In addition to everyone else
who came to the house
that scorching summer
our most regular visitor was
my mother's bestie Elaine
with her dog Henry
the smelliest shih tzu
in the entire world.

When I came home
Elaine's car was often
standing in the driveway.
Inside I found her
at the kitchen island
reading a newspaper
or solving a crossword
with Henry in her lap.

Sara would take me aside
and whisper quickly
'I didn't get much done
because Elaine showed up.'

Whereupon I assured Sara
that taking care of Elaine
was part of her job.

Now and then
Sara and Elaine and I
went out for breakfast.
We held on to each other
around the abyss of
my mother's absence.

Where was my mother?
Where was she?
We looked around
but all we saw
was each other.

Slowly Sara and I
emptied the house.

We gave away
hundreds of books
dozens of furniture items
hundreds of porcelain pieces
and 80 pairs of black trousers.

As the contents of
my mother's house
gradually vanished
Sara and I became
happier and lighter.

But at the same time
we also became
sadder and heavier.
As the house disappeared
so did my mother.
More space was created
for the fathomless void
she had left behind.

The house wasn't pregnant
with my mother's absence.
It was screaming.

**O**ne more thing
from that hot summer.

My mother often told me
that after she died
I would need a stylist
to furnish the house.
She even left a folder
with newspaper articles
on stylists in our area.

Patty the real estate agent
recommended a stylist
and one hot day
Patty and the woman
walked through the house
with Sara and me
to discuss the new decor.

Afterward Sara and I
stood together beside
the back window
that looked out onto
the lush backyard.
Suddenly Sara gasped
and pointed at the window.
'Look at that!'

A hummingbird!
Tiny and blue
floating in the air

a few inches
from the window.

Its wings flapped
incredibly fast
and its small eyes
stared fixedly at us.

The bird stayed a long time
observing Sara and me.
Then it flew away.

In all my life
I had never seen
a hummingbird in NJ.
I had also never seen
any bird whatsoever
remain still so long
and stare in that way.

Sara and I looked
at one another.
'My mother?'
I wondered aloud.

'I think so'
Sara replied.

The next day
I told this story
to my friend Jackie
and she turned pale.

Jackie said
'My grandfather died
at home in his bed.
The next day
when my mother
and grandmother
changed the sheets
they saw a hummingbird
outside the window
watching them.

'In all their decades
living in that house

they had never once
seen a hummingbird.

'It was obvious to them
the hummingbird
was my grandfather
who wanted to say
that he was OK.
Afterward my mother
got a hummingbird tattoo
to honor the moment.'

Well then.
My mother and I
had talked about
her contacting me
after her death.

'Do it if you can'
I told her.
'But nothing creepy!
Don't move furniture
or write messages
on mirrors.'

It was you mom!
A little bird
nimble and colorful
living among the flowers
in your fragrant backyard.

It was you mom!
Thanks for coming
and letting us know
that you were OK.


By mid-August
my mother's house
was emptied and styled
and ready for sale.

That was actually
several weeks earlier
than anticipated
due entirely to the

seamless teamwork
between Sara and me.

Our last task
was burying
a St. Joseph statue
in the front yard.
According to tradition
the statue would help
sell the house.

When I told Sara
I wanted to do this
she said it definitely
was worth a try.

I went on Amazon
where I bought
a St. Joseph packet
containing a little statue
and a brochure with
burial instructions
and a short prayer.

Sara and I carried out
the ceremony together.
We buried the statue
upside down
in the front yard
next to the large
FOR SALE sign.
We bowed our heads
and said the prayer.

Two weeks later
in Woodstock NY
at a backyard party
hosted by my friend Joan
my phone rang.
Patty the real estate agent
informed me that
someone wanted
to buy the house.

A boulder fell
off my chest.

It was the first time
that whole summer
I actually took
a full breath.

And the statue
of St. Joseph?
Did it actually
help sell the house?

I decided that
it didn't matter
if it was true.
The most important thing
was that it worked.


In May 2017
I had a mother
a dog and a cat
a home and an address.

By September 2017
everything was gone.

The life I had lived
with my mother
the previous four years
was now at an end.

Despite the very
occasional quarrel
and the sorrows of
the final months
those four years
were full of love
and much laughter.

But now everything
from that golden season
had disappeared.

Except for Sara.

I had lost
so much
but I still
had Sara.

# September 2017 to December 2018

The next 16 months
I lived alternatively
in NJ and Stockholm
with trips to Svalbard
(the Arctic archipelago
north of Norway)
to do research for
a new detective novel.

My goal was always
to find work in Sweden
but before I did that
I had to finalize
my mother's taxes
and other paperwork.
So now and then
I needed to travel
back to the US.

When I was in NJ
I didn't stay with Sara
because I wanted
to be in Westfield
with my yoga classes
and 12-step meetings.

I hired a room in
the center of Westfield
with a New Zealander
named Susannah and
her Siamese cat Rosie
who resembled
an elegant vampire
thanks to one very
long front tooth.

But even though
I lived in Westfield
Sara's home
felt like my home.

Imagine if your life
suddenly fell apart

and you had
no job
no home
no money.
Who would you
turn to then?

When my mother
was still alive
her house was
the place I could
always go back to.
My address and home
literally and emotionally.

Now that my mother
and her house were gone
Sara's house became
that place for me
literally and emotionally.

Partly because
Sara said so
but mostly because
it was obvious
and didn't need
to be said at all.

When I was in NJ
I often saw Sara
and Lucky.

Our meeting place
was the parking lot
behind Starbucks.
We bought coffee
then Sara drove us
to my mother's grave
in Fairview Cemetery.

The plot is under a tree
with a granite headstone.
My mother and father
and my sister Diane
are all buried there.

One day I probably
will be there too.

Sara and I
always brought
an extra black coffee
and poured it out
onto the grave.

We were sure
even death itself
had not shaken
the intense love
my mother had
for black coffee.

Think of it as
a liquid love letter
from Sara and me
and Lucky too.

**S**trangely enough
it was during a visit
to my mother's grave
Sara and I learned
that little Lucky
was seriously ill.

Sara and her family
had adopted Lucky and
he had adjusted himself
to a *new* new family.

Everyone loved Lucky
except their other dog
the blind white poodle
named Jordie.
Sara always said
Lucky and Jordie
got along well.
But later Little Sarah
said Jordie hated Lucky
and sometimes Jordie
even peed on him.

In any case.
One day Sara and I
were at the grave
without Lucky.
He had been unwell
so Vickie had taken him
to the local vet.

While Sara and I stood
at the gravesite and
spoke with my mother
Sara's phone rang.

Vickie said
the vet said
Lucky needed to go
to the emergency vet
immediately.

Sara and I left
and met Vickie at
the emergency vet
where we found out
Lucky had diabetes.
Which meant he needed
insulin shots twice a day
as well as special food
and regular blood tests.

I would have understood
if Sara and her family
had said to me then
'Adopting Lucky
hasn't turned out
like we imagined.
Can you possibly
take him back?'

I wouldn't have been
angry with them
even though
taking Lucky back
would have meant
I needed to stay
in Westfield

and make a home
for him and me.

But that conversation
never happened.
And that's because Sara
had promised my mother
to take care of Lucky.
They had made
a sacred pact.
End of discussion.

The rest of Sara's family
also wanted Lucky
despite his illness.
Sara's husband Frank
told me several times
'This dog will be loved
until the day he dies.'

Such fine people
make the world
gleam like gold.

After so many years
in so many places
Lucky had finally found
his final home.


During those months
when I was back in NJ
my friendship with Sara
entered a new phase.

We no longer had
an ailing mother
to keep alive
nor did we have
an overstuffed house
we needed to empty.

We ceased being
employer and employee
even though to me
it had always felt

like both of us
worked for my mother.

Now Sara and I
were just two women
who liked to hang out
and talk about our lives.

That's when Sara told me
that as a young girl in Brazil
it was never her dream
to immigrate to the US
but rather to Spain.
That was the place
Sara and her friends
dreamed about.

That's when Sara told me
how she met her husband
when she was in Brazil
and he was in America
and they wrote letters
for months before
meeting face to face.

We discussed Sara's
immigration to NJ.
First an apartment
in Newark
then a house
in Linden.

'That's the immigrant's journey'
she explained to me.
'You start in Newark
then move to a smaller city
and maybe later a suburb.'

Of course Sara and I
talked about my mother.
Things I knew and
things I didn't know.

For example
my mother told Sara
she worried about me

because I didn't have
a man in my life.

For example
whenever I came back
from traveling abroad
my mother always
announced to Sara
whether I had lost
or gained weight.

Those walks with Sara
were slow and peaceful
friendly and pleasant.
I enjoyed every single one
as did Sara and Lucky.


During one walk
Lucky rushed ahead
plopped on the ground
and rolled in goose poop
thick oily and green.

Sara's method
for handling this
was 100 percent Sara.

She laughed and
took Lucky to her car
where she rinsed him off
with bottles of water
then dried him carefully
with paper towels.

In the midst of dealing
with the green poop
reams of dirty paper
and wet smelly Lucky
Sara looked at me
and declared calmly
'If you have a dog
you have to expect
things like this.'

To which I would add
if you have a friend

like my Sara
you learn to expect
kind and gentle
reactions like that.

In so many ways
Sara was my role model.


**A**nother thing
Sara and I did
whenever I was
back in Westfield
was drive by
my mother's house.

A drive-by
as it's called.

The house was situated
between downtown
and the cemetery
so we did a drive-by
almost every time
we met for a walk.

As Sara inched
past the house
we called out
all the little changes
the new family had made.

It was a pleasure
to see the house
but also a sorrow
because my mother
wasn't there and
we couldn't go inside.

One day when
we did a drive-by
the new family
was outside.

The son was
playing basketball
with a new hoop.

The mother was
pruning the hedges
by the front door.

The father was
working on a project
in the garage.

Sara and I drove by
quickly that day
not wanting to attract
the new family's attention.

That was the moment
I truly understood
the house belonged
to someone else.

That was the moment
I finally realized
it was time to let go
of my mother's house.

By some kind
of silent agreement
Sara and I never did
a drive-by again.


In August 2018
my mother's estate
finally was finalized.

I went back
to Stockholm
with no plan
to return to NJ.

During the months
I was in Sweden
Sara and I spoke
every few weeks.
I missed her and
my other friends
but I no longer
had a home in NJ

and it felt barren
without my mother.

Sara knew my goal
was to establish
a life in Sweden.
She believed in my dream
and she encouraged me.

The only thing
Sara wanted for me
was for me
to be happy.

Sunday December 23 2018
5:45 pm.

Christmas lights
twinkled throughout
coal-black Stockholm.

My 90 tourist days
in Sweden were
about to run out.
On Christmas Day
I would travel
to Copenhagen
then fly over to
the Faroe Islands
for a 12-step convention.

Afterward I would
travel to Svalbard
for an artist's residency
to write my detective novel.
Then back to Sweden
where I planned to
find full-time work
and live there for
the rest of my life.

I stood in
Central Station
in the ticket office
a large lively room
with several clerks

behind counters.
I was in the area where
you could sit or stand
and wait for someone
to call out your number.

Why did I call Sara
from Central Station?

I don't remember.
Probably because
I had promised
to get in touch
at a certain time
and I wasn't yet
back at my hotel
namely Freys Hotel
which I knew about
from reading
Stieg Larsson's
The Girl Who
Played with Fire.

I stood in a quiet corner
took out my phone
and called Sara.


Vickie answered.

That was odd.
Sometimes Sara
handed her phone
over to Vickie
so Vickie could explain
something to me
which Sara had trouble
expressing in English.
But Vickie never
answered Sara's phone.

'Hey Vickie!
Is everything OK?'

'Hey Florence.
Everything's all right.

But my mother is
in the hospital.'

Vickie told me that
two days earlier
Sara had a seizure.
They brought her
to the hospital and
she had two more.

Tests were done.
An MRI showed
several tumors
in Sara's brain.

She needed more tests
and maybe an operation
in order to determine
if the tumors were
benign or malignant.

Central Station
vanished briefly.

When it came back
the lights were
too strong
the sounds were
too harsh.

The background
and foreground
changed places
several times.

My eardrums filled
with the frenetic flapping
of the sorrow bird's wings.

That was the moment
life broke in two.

It wasn't the first time
that happened to me.
And it wasn't always
something bad

although sometimes
like now
it was.

1973 when I got
my first period.

1980 when I was accepted
to Barnard College.

1990 when I moved
to a small village in Crete.

1991 when my nephew
Alexander was born.

1995 when I left Crete
and my husband.

1996 when my niece
Flora was born.

2006 when my boyfriend
Taikyu rolled away on
an escalator at JFK airport.

2010 when my sister Diane died.

2013 when my father died.

2017 when my mother died.

And now again
Stockholm Central Station
December 2018.

One of those moments
when life breaks
into two pieces
a before and an after.

And what was before
never comes back.


It happened like this.

December 20 2018
in the afternoon
Sara decided to buy
Christmas sweaters

for Lucky and Jordie.
That errand describes
Sara to a tee.

Sara drove Frank and
Little Sarah to TJ Maxx.
She bought the sweaters
and they returned to the car.

Sara was driving them
out of the parking lot
when something happened
when it happened.

Later Sara told me
the seizure felt as if
someone was holding
a vacuum-cleaner nozzle
against her cheek.

Later Little Sarah told me
she knew immediately
something was wrong
because Sara stopped talking
in the middle of a sentence.
(Sara are you still talking?)

They drove Sara
to the hospital
and that's where
they got the news
about the tumors
in Sara's brain.


When I called Sara
from Central Station
it was two days later.

Sara had been
in the hospital
the entire time
with Vickie at her side
the entire time
even at night.

'Can I talk
to your mom?'
I asked Vickie.

'Sure' she said.

Sara's musical
Brazilian accent
was a little hoarse
but warm as always.
'Hello my dear!'

My throat thickened.
I stammered
'Vickie told me
what happened.'

In a tranquil voice
Sara replied
'They'll find out
what's wrong
and then I'll get
treatment for it.'

Her words
helped me
calm down
a little.

Sara was right.
It was just a matter
of getting information
and then doing
whatever was needed.

It was OK.
People got brain tumors.
It happened.

But still.
Brain tumors.
And so many?


We talked as
I stood stock-still
in the ticket room
of Central Station

with dozens of people
moving around me.

I clung to Sara's voice
as shock cascaded
through my senses
and dismantled reality
as I had known it.

As we spoke
the wall between
before and after
was being erected
at lightning speed.

Just as soon as
the wall was finished
the sorrow bird
perched on the edge
with inconsolable eyes
and watched as Sara
started to disappear.

# Part 2

# Sara Disappears

# 2018–2020

Christmas 2018.
On the train
to Copenhagen.

I like to travel
on Christmas Day.
Empty cities possess
a quiet magic.

As soon as I arrived
at my hotel room
next to Central Station
I called Sara.

Few people I knew
loved Christmas
as much as Sara.
It was unbearable
to think of my friend
in the hospital
on just that day.

As Sara's phone rang
I steeled myself
for the conversation
on its way.

Sara answered
at once.
'Hello my dear!'

I asked how
she was doing
and Sara told me
she was home.

A stone fell
off my heart.
Sara was home!
With her family
and her dogs
and her friends
and her Christmas!
Everyone
and everything
she loved.

Relief spread
through me.
My fear eased
a little bit.

Sara was home!
If the doctors
sent her home
things couldn't be
so terribly bad.
Right?

As the wise Dean
once stated:
Home is home.

Sara also told me
her doctor had decided
to operate and remove
the biggest tumor.

A tissue analysis
would reveal
the true nature
of the growths.

Sara didn't use
the word cancer
but I understood
what she didn't say.

The operation
was scheduled
for mid-January.
Until then Sara
had nothing to do
except enjoy Christmas
with her family
and friends
and cherished dogs.

OK.
Not OK at all
but OK.

We had gotten
a little reprieve.

I wished Sara
Merry Christmas
then said goodbye.

# Winter to Spring 2019

A week later
January 2019.

Time to begin
my artist residency
in the archipelago
of Svalbard
famed for its
brutal landscape
roaming polar bears
five months of
constant sunlight
five months of
constant darkness.

I had spent time
in the village of
Longyearbyen
during different
seasons of the year
but this would be
my first visit in
the dark season.

When I arrived
I had a violent cold
and was still shaky
after a visa problem
which could have led
to a large fine or
expulsion from Europe
for one year.

I had thought
the art gallery
where I was staying
would be full of people
both the little hostel
on the second floor
and the gallery and
artist workshops
on the bottom floor.

But no.
Christmas break
in Norway is long
so the gallery
was closed
and the workshops
were empty.

The only guest
in the hostel
and the only artist
doing a residency
was me.

Just like that
I was sick and weak
alone and isolated
in the darkest darkness
on the planet
except of course
the earth's other pole
Antarctica.

The village was
long and thin.

Steep mountains
imprisoned it
on both sides.

Avalanches were
a looming danger.
Just a few years before
an avalanche had
killed a child and
injured nine others.

Ice coated the roads
making each step
fraught with peril
since it was not
possible to detect
ice in the darkness.

Everyone promised me
polar bears never came

into the village itself.
That was good to hear
but on a previous visit
I had a close encounter
with a polar bear
which left a terror
deep in my soul
impossible to extinguish.

Polar bears
don't hibernate.
Even in winter's
incessant blackout
they are still awake
and on the move.
That fact was also
impossible to forget.

And the birds?
Winter in Svalbard
was too cold for them.
The only exception
was the sorrow bird
whose favorite color
was darkness.

Worst of all
I literally couldn't
leave Svalbard.

Exiting the archipelago
required traveling
through Norway.
Due to the problem
with my visa
I had used up
all my tourist days
so I didn't have
even one extra day
for the obligatory
stopover in Norway.

As soon as I arrived
in Longyearbyen
I wanted to leave

but I had to wait
90 more days
in the bleak and
constant nighttime
until my visa clock
finally reset.

The darkness
was immoveable
and I couldn't move
away from it.

Then there was Sara.
Being overseas
when she was ill
added another
layer of darkness.

Even though Svalbard
was extremely remote
the internet connection
was thankfully strong
and I spoke to Sara
several times before
her impending operation.

During one call
Sara said she decided
to shave her own head
instead of waiting
for nurses to do it
the day of her operation.

'Good!' I said.
'That makes it
your decision
and your choice.'

We realized that
even though Sara
had lost control
over so many
aspects of her life
there were still things

she could decide
for herself.

That became a question
we turned over
again and again
like a Zen koan:
What did Sara still
have control over?

Our conversations
were full of warmth
and as usual I enjoyed
chatting with Sara.

But every time
we said goodbye
and my room in
the empty hostel
filled with silence
I started crying.

Sara my Sara!
It tore me apart
to see my friend
imprisoned in
this waking nightmare.

**A** few days before
Sara's surgery
I googled the term
brain tumor.

Like everyone else
I googled constantly
but I had avoided
just that phrase.

What a relief
when I found out
most brain tumors
are benign.

I decided to assume
Sara's tumors
were also benign.

My heart lightened
a tiny bit.

Now I had a strategy
for going forward.
A little boat
to sit still in
while I waited
all alone in
an empty building
in a dark village
in the pitiless Arctic.

The operation
went well.

The lab began
analyzing the tissue.
Sara promised to call
as soon as the doctor
gave her the results.

A few days passed
with no word
from Sara or Vickie.

I got worried
and called them.

No answer.

The next afternoon
after lunch at Rabalder
one of Longyearbyen's
few restaurants
my phone rang.

Vickie.

I left Rabalder and
stood in the wide hallway
just outside the restaurant
in the little shopping center.

I answered but
Vickie didn't
say anything.

She was crying.
Just crying.

A cold hand
circled my heart.
No I thought.
No no no.

Vickie couldn't
bear to say
what needed
to be said
so I decided
to say it for her.
'You got bad news.'

In spaces between
gut-wrenching sobs
Vickie told me
that Sara had
aggressive brain cancer
with a maximum of
two years left to live.

She added that
some people with
this type of cancer
survived up to five years.

Vickie told me
the cancer's name:
glioblastoma.

She said that Sara
couldn't bear
to give me the news.
I understood that
because I knew
that Sara knew
how much this truth
would destroy me.

Once again
I had gotten

horrific news
in a public space.

There I stood
in a hallway
outside a restaurant
in a shopping center
in a little village
deep in the Arctic.

People walked past
encased in thick jackets
furry hats with earflaps
faces red from the cold
laughing and speaking
Norwegian and Russian.
Every one of them
was a stranger.

Although I was inside
the hall was not well-lit
especially in the corners.
The darkness outside
was so impenetrable
that indoors never felt
truly light either.

As I stood
in the weak light
the sorrow bird
began to sing
a black song
frantic and feverish
bitter and cold.


**M**y sister Diane died
in 2010.

My father died
in 2013.

My mother died
in 2017.

I had assumed
Death would

leave me in peace
at least for a while.

Apparently not.


The news that Sara
had aggressive brain cancer
would have devastated me
no matter where I was.

But finding out about it
while isolated in a dark and
dangerous corner of the world
was a special sort of hell.

When my conversation
with Vickie was over
I plodded numbly
up the frozen hill
into the empty hostel
in the deserted gallery.

I got on Skype
and called Joanna
my 12-step sponsor
who lived in NJ.
She listened with
deep compassion
and helped me manage
the first bottomless shock.

But the moment came
when I had to hang up
and was forced to bear
my unbearable feelings
alone.

In the middle of
the Arctic darkness
the sorrow bird sang
an icy hymn
pulsating with pain.


I talked with Sara
a few days later

and after that we spoke
once or twice a week.

It was always a comfort
to hear her voice.
'Hello my dear!'

Sara was alive!
Yes she was sick
yes she had cancer
aggressive and incurable
but just that moment
she was alive.

I hadn't lost Sara.
Not yet.

But at the same time
everything was different.
I listened with
a grieving heart
as Sara updated me
on her condition.

Sara's treatment
wasn't going well.
Her white-blood cells
had plummeted to
the same level as
someone with AIDS.

The doctor ordered
Sara to stay home
in order to avoid
picking up an infection.

Overnight
Sara's life
became small.
She no longer drove
nor did she work
go shopping
or meet friends.
She was only allowed
to leave the house

for doctor visits
and treatments.

Note this was 2019.
Being ordered
to stay at home
to avoid infection
was a strange and
foreign concept.

Sara was alone
in being home
alone.

Gradually I realized
Sara didn't want
to discuss her illness.
She could do that
with her doctors.

From me Sara needed
laughter and small talk
and our favorite topic
my mother.

We talked about
my mother's unique language
such as calling Facebook
Spacebook.

We talked about
my mother's peculiar logic
which included
her plan to downsize
via buying an enormous
flat-screen TV
that she never learned
how to turn on.

We talked about
my mother's big heart
and all the charities
she supported
which ranged from
operations for children
with cleft palates

to a special shelter
for homeless rabbits.

These memories
were our way
of traveling back
to a time and life
not so long ago.
A time when
my mother was alive
Sara was healthy
and Lucky was too.

Those conversations
gave me a lifeline
a way out of being
stuck in a room
in a dark village
in one of the world's
most desolate places
where every step outside
was life-threatening.

I imagine our phone calls
felt the same for Sara.
She also was trapped
inside her house
and every step outside
was life-threatening.
Living in a body with
aggressive brain cancer
was surely one of the most
dark and desolate places
a human could experience.

O Sara!
Sara my Sara.

Talking with Sara
soothed me
and hopefully
comforted her.

At the same time
I longed to do

something concrete
to help her cope.

Once a week
I sent a postcard
with a picture of
Svalbard's wildlife
foxes and puffins
walruses and dolphins
polar bears and reindeer.

Sara loved animals and
I hoped my postcards
brought her joy.
But still they felt
insufficient.
Surely there was more
I could do for her.

One day I decided
to send Sara flowers
(and read later that
you shouldn't give
flowers to cancer patients
because the petals
might contain bacteria).

Another day I decided
to send Sara a check
to help out financially
(and two weeks later
got a call from
an embarrassed Vickie
who told me that
the bank had refused
to accept the check
because I had written
the numbers so sloppily).

How I longed
to fix this for Sara!
There had to be
some way to make
the unbearable bearable.

That powerlessness
roared like hunger
burned like thirst
every bleak day
in the darkness.

**H**owever
I did do one thing
that seemed to work.

When I was 42
I had a serious crisis.
My addictions had
taken over my life.
I was lost and unhappy
and wanted desperately
to reawaken my good heart.

Although I wasn't Catholic
I started attending
St. Francis of Assisi Church
in Manhattan.
I also bought the book
Novena: The Power of Prayer.
(A novena is a prayer
you direct toward
a particular saint and
repeat for nine days.)

That's when I discovered
St. Therese of Lisieux
otherwise known as
Little Therese or
Therese of the Little Flower
who before her death
solemnly declared
'I want to spend my heaven
doing good on earth.'

For nine days
I prayed fervently
to Little Therese.

It's said that when
Little Therese has

heard your prayer
roses will appear
in some way.
So I started keeping
an eye out for roses.

On the Sunday morning
after I had completed
my nine days of prayer
I emerged from
Port Authority Bus Terminal
in Manhattan
to go to my job at
a soulless law firm.
That's when I saw
strewn across the sidewalk
dozens of red rose petals.

Dumbstruck
I stopped short.
Could it be?
No way!
It was impossible.

Later that day
I was sent to work
at another desk.
When I arrived
there was a vase
on the desk with
a lovely bouquet
of white roses.

Dumbstruck again.
Could it be?
No way!
It was impossible.

Or maybe
it was possible
after all?

That was when
my heart united with
Little Therese's heart.

In any case
that's how it felt.

Not long afterward
Buddhism became
my spiritual life
and so it remained
for many years.

Once in a while
I remembered
Little Therese
and when I did
I always thought
about those roses.

Now it was 2018.
I was stuck in Svalbard
and my best friend
was terminally ill.

One day in the hostel
I paced the floor
desperate to find
a way to help Sara.

I realized I needed
spiritual help.
Time to call on
the A-team.
Time to petition
a truly powerful saint.

Suddenly Little Therese
popped up in my heart.

Little Therese!
Of course.
I remembered the roses
and the burning promise
she made before her death.

Google led me to
an organization called
Society of the Little Flower
in Darien IL.

I ordered a mass
in Sara's name and
the Society promised
to conduct the mass
and afterward send
a mass card to Sara.

I knew about mass cards
because I received one
when Elaine ordered
a mass for my mother
after her death.

Obviously
this was a long shot.
I didn't even know
if Sara was religious.
We never discussed it
and I couldn't recall
Sara ever mentioning
attending church.

But if there was
any chance at all
there truly was
a positive energy
called Little Therese
I had to at least try.

**A** few weeks later
Sara told me
she had received
the mass card.

'Great' I said.

'But Florence'
she replied
'do you know
my middle name?'

'No' I said.

'My middle name
is Terezinha.
Little Therese.
I was named after her.'

A thousand rose petals
danced through my room
and sparkled with joy.

During my three months
confined in Svalbard
I had a routine.

Every morning
after writing
I left the hostel
and ventured outside
into the ruthless cold
and bitter darkness.

I swaddled myself in
long underwear
woolen slacks
an Icelandic sweater
long down jacket
reflective vest
chunky socks
boots with spikes
hat with earflaps
under my coat hood
lined in fake fur.

As I inched my way
down the icy road
to Longyearbyen's center
I counted days
aloud to myself.
How many days
I had been there
and how many days
I still had left.

The number of
remaining days
fell slowly
one by one.
That minuscule
decrease in time
afforded me

enough relief
to keep going.

In any case
forward to
the next breath.

Look!
A middle-aged woman
from Westfield NJ
trapped within
perpetual midnight
trudges along a road
in a hostile place
she doesn't want to be
but isn't allowed to leave.

Look!
A middle-aged woman
with a heavy heart
takes comfort from
counting days
alone in the dark.


Then and
maybe now
Longyearbyen had
no 12-step meetings
no yoga studio
nothing I needed
in order to maintain
my emotional balance.

My best friend was ill
and my mental state
was precarious.

The constant darkness
pressed against me
like a living creature
smothering me
inside and out
leaving me in
a perpetual state
of suffocation.

In order to dampen
the black song
of the sorrow bird
I worked constantly.
My writing life
kept me aloft
as did frequent
online Swedish lessons
with my kind teacher Óren.

Occasionally
glimmers of light
illuminated my life
in Longyearbyen.

One dark morning
someone held
a restorative yoga class
in a closed hotel.
A one-time thing
but it lit an inner light
that helped me go forward.

In any case
forward to
the next breath.

I even made
several friends.
Marie the librarian
Ingeborg the gallerist
the PhD students
Magda and Molly and Sarah.

One problem with
my new friendships
was that I didn't want
any of them to see
how unhappy I was.
Life in Svalbard
was hard for everyone
and I didn't want
to be negative.

My friends never knew
that I promised myself

every single day
to never *never* NEVER
return to Svalbard
as soon as I finally
was free to leave.

One person
who I did tell
was the village's
lone therapist
a Brazilian woman
named Anna.

Once a week
on the second floor
of the shopping center
I crawled into her office
in a thousand pieces
and opened my heart.
I was drowning
and she was kind.

Just as I sent
Sara postcards
of beautiful wildlife
to offer a little light
so did the Universe
send me kind people
to help me survive
the piercing darkness.

At least
that's how it felt.


**I** had another project
to occupy my time
while I was in Svalbard.

My mother's estate
had finally wrapped up
and at last I was able
to search for work
in Stockholm.

I unearthed my resume
from my laptop.

I joined LinkedIn
and applied for jobs.

But at the same time
the longing to be
with my Sara in NJ
kept growing stronger.

Sara was beginning
a difficult journey
of uncertain length
and I wanted to be
right by her side.

From my mother's
decline and death
I knew that Sara
and her family
were going to need
every bit of help
they could possibly get.

I also knew that
during the years
with my mother
when I postponed
my move to Sweden
it often felt like
my obligations
weighed me down
and crushed my dreams.

A hellish tug-of-war:
My mother or me?
Duty or freedom?

Now I was there again.
Conflicting thoughts
wrestled one another
in my head
in my heart.

And then
just like that
during a dark walk

to the village center
something shifted.

All at once
my soul decided
to return to NJ.
Not that
I had to go back.
Rather that
I wanted to.

I would wait out
my remaining time
in Svalbard
then go to Stockholm
to launch my book
The Grand Man.

After that
I would go to NJ
to be with Sara
and help her out
until the end.

I set my dream
of Sweden on ice
and saved my resume
in a file called
Miscellaneous.

The inner battle
had gone quiet.
My heart could
finally exhale.

The sorrow bird
lowered its head
folded its wings
and prepared to wait.

Another ray of light
was that Sara
was still Sara.

The one time
I googled

glioblastoma
I discovered that
personality changes
often occurred
during the course
of the illness.

Every time
Sara and I talked
I was alert to
what she said and
how she said it.

It was always a relief
to hear that Sara
was still Sara.

It felt like I had
a bit of time
despite everything.
I was sure that
it would be OK
to stay overseas
a few more months.

Sara still
was Sara.
She wasn't so sick
even though
she was dying.

Two months
into my residency
the sun came back
to Longyearbyen.

It was a slow process.
First came
the blue season
with several hours
of twilight.

Then came
the pink season
with several hours
of sunrise.

More light yes
but still no sun.

Finally on March 8
the village gathered
to welcome the sun
as it emerged over
a craggy mountaintop
at 12.50 pm.

I stood with Marie
by the red wooden church
jumping up and down
to warm ourselves
chanting loudly
with the others
'Sun sun come again
the sun is my best friend!'

When the bright yellow light
peeked over the mountaintop
euphoria glistened
through my every cell.

I had been longing
for just that sunrise
during each dark moment
of my time in Svalbard.

Unfortunately
there was a catch.
The sun came up
but after 15 minutes
it went down again.

I had forgotten
about that part.

Afterward
I went inside the church
with the rest of the village
and ate crispy waffles
smothered in jam and
fresh whipped cream.

Walking home
I felt terribly sad.

I wasn't prepared for
how it would feel
when the sun once again
left me in the dark.

# Spring 2019

Finally Stockholm!

Bright spring light
coffee with friends
yoga and 12-step meetings.

Majestic buildings
reflecting from
the glittering water.

The cherry blossoms
of Kungsträdgården
gloriously in bloom.

The exquisite sound
of the Swedish language
dancing in the air.

Nonetheless
as I strolled around
springtime Stockholm
delighted by the light
and lack of polar bears
I could still hear
all the way from NJ
the sorrow bird's ballad.

I had been freed
while Sara remained
imprisoned in her home
by her white blood cells.

I mourned for my friend
who couldn't step outside
and join the newborn world
shimmering with spring.


In the middle of
spring in Stockholm
I traveled to France.

Not for vacation
but rather a pilgrimage

to find Little Therese
in Lisieux.

The conversation
I had with Sara
when she told me
her middle name
felt like a sign.
After that
I started praying
every single day
to Little Therese.

Many people say
it doesn't work
if you pray directly
for what you want
so I didn't dare.
My prayers were
always unassuming
just a timid little
'Please help Sara.'

Gradually I got tired
of being cautious.
I wanted to ask Therese
to heal Sara completely.
I wanted to dare!

The idea of making
a pilgrimage to Lisieux
to say this prayer
rose up within me
several times a day
and would not let go.

Does it sound ludicrous?
Maybe so.
But when Sara was gone
I wanted to look back
and know I had done
everything in my power
to help her heal.

That included
looking for help

from someone
or something
with real power
and by that I mean
spiritual power.

And why not?
Sara wanted to live.
During one of our
many phone calls
she had burst out
'I want to live!'

Those words stabbed me
and echoed mercilessly.

It wasn't like that
for my mother
who declared
'I don't know why
I'm still here.'

Different songs from
two dying women.
Both of those melodies
broke my heart.

April 2019
I flew from Stockholm to Paris
hailed a taxi to Gare Saint-Lazare
took a train to Lisieux.

I don't speak French
and during my journey
I felt lost and confused.
It certainly didn't help
that everyone I met
refused to speak English
even the man who worked
at the information booth
in the train station.

But so what!
My heart was on fire.
If I needed to
I would crawl

the 98 miles
from Paris to Lisieux.

Nothing and nobody
was going to stop me
from saying my prayer.

Finally Lisieux.

A long walk from
the train station
to my hotel
in the city center.

Lisieux is not
a charming city
but it's an important one
because once upon a time
it nurtured a saint.

Therese's family moved
to Lisieux in 1877
when she was 4
and Therese lived there
until her death at 24.

Among bland buildings
rundown cafés and
fast food restaurants
several places remain
that were essential parts
of Little Therese's short life
such as her family home
her confirmation cathedral
and her nunnery.

There is also a basilica.
An enormous church
that holds 4000 people
built after Therese's death
to honor her memory.
It looks like the Taj Mahal
and is a strange site
in a modest French city.

**I** spent the afternoon
walking around the city
clutching a shiny map
that showed the places
connected to Little Therese.

I located each one
so I could come back
the next day and
chose a location
for my prayer.

The last place I went
was the nunnery office
so I could order
a mass for my Sara.

I stepped inside
the modest office
prepared to wrestle
with yet another
unpleasant person.

Mais non!
The French woman
at the reception desk
was kind and helpful
the very first person
willing to talk to me
since I had stepped
off the plane in Paris.

Her kindness
opened my heart
and when it was time
to open my mouth
the sorrow bird
flew out and sang
a long sad song.

I hadn't realized
the sorrow bird
was a ventriloquist.

The French woman
listened attentively

as I spoke to her
about my Sara.
My eyes filled
and my voice shook
as I shared everything
I had been carrying
since the day I stood
in Central Station
and life broke in two.

When I told the woman
the strange story of
Sara's middle name
she nodded calmly
as if she had heard
stories like mine
many times before.

I ordered the mass
and left the convent
with a sense of peace.
I had checked off
something essential
and in the bargain found
a compassionate witness
to my boundless pain.

The next morning
between stops in cafés
for bitter espresso
and buttery croissants
I visited the remains
of Little Therese's life.

Her childhood home
Les Buissonnets
was particularly moving.
I stood in the center
of Little Therese's room
which is where she had
a spiritual experience
at 12 years old
when she was deathly ill.

It was in that room
Therese pleaded for help
with all her heart and
it was in that room
she was healed.

The story gave me hope
but not entirely.
And that's because
a dozen years later
Little Therese died
from tuberculosis.
She had surely
prayed fervently
that time as well.
As did her family
and the other nuns.

Which left me
with a question:
Does prayer work?

To put it another way:
Is the Universe malleable?
If you press on it with
your thoughts and wishes
does it give way?

Sometimes it feels like that.
Sometimes not.

And if the Universe
isn't malleable?
Does that mean
everything is stuck
and already decided?

Sometimes it feels like that.
Sometimes not.

That was my question
during my days in Lisieux.
I never got an answer
or any inner clarity.

My only conclusion
was that Sara's illness

was not a time
when it was better
to be safe than sorry.
Rather I knew
I would be sorry
if I played it safe.

If there was any chance
I could help Sara
through prayer
I needed to grab
that invisible lifeline
and hold it tight
in my trembling hands.

Little Therese's basilica
was not for me.
I took a look inside
but it was far too big much
too extravagant.

Still it was remarkable that
the noble heart
of a young French girl had
inspired this building. And
even more amazing that
people had journeyed from
all over the world
in order to find her.

Because it wasn't just me
wandering around Lisieux
that muggy spring day. The
city overflowed
with eager pilgrims
clutching shiny maps
their faces glowing
with peace and faith.

The basilica had
a large gift shop
filled to the brim
with lovely objects
as well as Little Therese's
famous autobiography

The Story of a Soul
in dozens of languages.

I wanted to buy
the book for Sara
but I couldn't figure out
the difference between
Spanish and Portuguese
and it was Portuguese
Sara needed.

Due to the chilly reception
I had thus far received
(with the exception of
the lady at the nunnery)
I wanted to avoid
asking for help.
In France
my American accent
was my worst enemy.

But this was important
so I went up to a clerk
a young woman
tall and thin with
long brown hair and
soulful brown eyes
and asked her for help.

When the woman heard
my American song
her eyes lit up
just like eyes
light up in Sweden
where everyone is eager
to speak English.

As it turned out
the young woman
was engaged
to an American
and was planning
to move to Ohio.

She told me that
she was in Lisieux

working in the gift shop
because she had had
certain experiences
with Little Therese
and wanted to be
closer to her.

Such a welcoming person
was exactly what I needed.

I didn't refer to
my Sara by name
but I said a friend
was seriously ill
and I was in Lisieux
to pray for her.

Just like the woman
at the nunnery office
the young woman
nodded calmly
as if she had heard
such stories
many times before.

She found the right book
and I thanked her.
I said I planned
to return to the shop
the next morning
before I left for Paris.

'Please do!' she said.
'I'll be here.'

In that hostile land
it finally felt
like I had a friend.


In the afternoon
I went to the cathedral
where Little Therese
had been confirmed.

A gray stone building
900 years old

shadowy and still
with a soaring ceiling
and dozens of nooks
to light a candle
and say a prayer.

I walked softly
in that peaceful space
until I stopped at
a black-iron candelabra
standing in view of
a stained-glass window.

I lit a candle
and knelt down
on the kneeling pad
in front of a statue
of Little Therese.

This was what
I had come for.
It was time.

I said aloud
'Little Therese!
Please take away
Sara's cancer.
But if you can't
for some reason
I don't understand
and probably never will
because I have no idea
how the Universe works
please help Sara
get through this.
Don't abandon her.
And by the way
please help me
to help her.
Thank you.'

I stayed silent
a few more breaths.
Then I rose up

and brushed off
my dusty knees.

At last I had done
what needed doing.
To pray
for a miracle.
To allow room
for a miracle.

And why not?
It never hurts to ask
and you don't lose
anything by trying.

As I mentioned
I don't know how
the Universe works
but I did know
my own heart.
That pilgrimage
and that prayer
was something
I had to do
and at last
it was done.

The remainder of
my time in Lisieux
went slowly.

I walked around
indifferent to
the charmless city.
Now that my prayer
had been said
all I wanted
was to leave.

I called Sara.
She knew I had
gone to Lisieux
although I never
told her why.

I ordered Chinese food
and watched a film
in my hotel room
with its saggy bed
and retro wallpaper
featuring a lavish design
of colossal orange flowers.

I was tired and
the sorrow bird
sung in French
which meant
I understood
nothing at all.

It's said you know
when Little Therese
has heard your prayer
because roses appear
in some way.

The moment I left
the majestic cathedral
I was on the lookout
for my roses.

But no.
I didn't see
one single rose
not even a petal
during the remainder
of my time in Lisieux.

There was however
one surprise
waiting for me.

My final morning
I went back
to the gift shop
at the basilica
to buy presents for
Sara and her family
and other friends.

I had another chat
with the young clerk
who was just as kind
as the day before.

I gathered together
my shiny gifts
and paid for them.

On the way out
I went over to
the young woman
and thanked her
for all the help.

'By the way' I said
'My name is Florence.'

She smiled and said
'My name is Sara.'

A shock of delight
coursed through me.
My heart opened
like a rose bursting
into full bloom.

Was that the flower
I had been waiting for?

**O** Little Therese!
You did not remove
Sara's cancer
despite the fact
I implored you from
the very bottom
of my broken heart.

Rose petals did not
rain over me.

And yet
I don't regret
going to Lisieux.
It helped me
to try to help.

And who knows?
Maybe my pilgrimage
did comfort Sara
in some invisible way
that I don't understand.

In any case
that's what I hope.


**B**ack in Stockholm
I launched my book
and talked with Sara
every week.

One day in May
I phoned Elaine.
Now and then
I gave her a call
but this time
her number
was suspended.

My fingers shook
as I rang her brother.
I had never spoken
to him before but
I had asked Elaine
for his number
so I would be prepared
for exactly this situation.

Sure enough
Elaine had died
a few weeks before.
She had gone to a party
in her neighborhood
then came home
and had a heart attack
that same evening.

It warmed my heart
to hear that Elaine
was at a party
before she died.
Elaine loved to party!

And what about Henry
the smelliest shih tzu
in the entire world?

A few years before
Elaine had told me
'I pray every day
Henry dies before me
so I can nurse him
when he's dying
and so he won't
be left all alone
after I'm gone.'

Her prayer came true.
Henry died a year
before Elaine did.
She never got a new dog
but instead visited
a local animal shelter
to pet dogs there.

Elaine!
If Rosie's Wine Bar
has a branch in heaven
you and my mother
are sitting there now
with the many dogs
you both loved
during your long and
excellent lives.


Spring in Stockholm!
The majestic city sparkled
in the exquisite spring light.

A bittersweet beauty
because my return to NJ
loomed closer with
no firm date for
a return to Sweden.

But that was OK.
I wanted to be
with my Sara.

And thank goodness
whenever we spoke
Sara still
was Sara.
A little tired but
always full of love.

There was even good news!
Sara was no longer
imprisoned in her home.
She sent me pictures
from her first day outside
when Vickie and Little Sarah
drove her to a local park
filled with spring flowers.

In the pictures
Sara wore a big smile
large sunglasses
and a flowered scarf
wrapped elegantly
around her head.

Her entire being was
luminous with joy
radiant with sunlight.

One Monday evening
in early June
I called Sara
from Stockholm.

I was in Mariatorget
a lovely square with
a big fountain and
colorful flower beds.
I was on my way
to a 12-step meeting
and decided to give
Sara a quick call.

Immediately
I could hear
she was different.

I walked slowly among
the vibrant flower beds
and listened anxiously
as Sara spoke.
She talked slowly
with a low voice
and her words were
slightly slurred.

Suddenly Sara
gave the phone
to Vickie.

In a steady voice
Vickie told me
that her mother
didn't feel well
and would prefer
if we could talk
another day.

I went to my meeting
and shared about Sara
crying as I spoke.

The meeting helped but
afterward I was still sad.

Most of all I was
angry at myself.
When I left Svalbard
why didn't I return
directly to NJ?
I shouldn't have bothered
with the book launch
and the trip to Lisieux!

The future that
I had been dreading
was already here.


**A** few days before
I traveled back
to Westfield
I ate breakfast with

my friend Alise
at Bank Hotel.

I told her about
Sara's illness.
I said I was scared
to go back and
meet this new Sara.
I was afraid of
entering the storm
awaiting me there.

Alise said that
two of her friends
had been diagnosed
with breast cancer
and she had helped
both of them
up until the end.

'It'll be hard'
Alise told me
'but be sure
to keep an eye out
for the gifts.'

I stared at her.
'The gifts?'

Alise nodded.
'Because' she said
'there will be gifts.'

The rest of the day
I turned over
Alise's words
like pieces in
an intricate puzzle.

Was it possible that
the sorrow bird's cry
contained gifts?

The only way to find out
was to fly to the US
and plunge into
cancer's hurricane.

# Summer 2019

June 2019
once again
in Westfield.

Westfield was not
a bad place
but it never felt
like my place.

The only reason
I moved back in 2013
was to help my mother.
Now I was here again
this time to help Sara.

As usual I stayed
in the town center
in the apartment with
Susannah the New Zealander
and Rosie the Siamese
with the long front tooth.
My home in Westfield
since my mother's death.

I fell back
into my old life.
Friends
yoga studio
12-step meetings.
A simple life in
a simple suburb.

Being back in NJ
was comforting
but also confusing
since I had already
said goodbye.


The first time
Sara and I met up
that summer in NJ
was at Mindowaskin Park
in the center of Westfield.

A lush Saturday in June
a perfect summer day
comfortably warm
with a light breeze.

The park was alive
with tall leafy trees
blooming flower beds
and families of ducks
gliding on the long pond.

In the center was
a wooden pavilion
where once as a teenager
I danced hand in hand
with a handsome boy
in a black high hat.
Another world
in a different time.

Sara and Little Sarah
sat on a bench
waiting for me.
Sara looked beautiful
with a silk scarf
wound around her head
and that big smile.

'Hello my dear!'
she exclaimed.

We hugged.
Ten months
had passed
and finally
I was back.

Nonetheless I was
full of trepidation.
Our last conversation
in Stockholm
echoed anxiously
in my heart.

To my delight
Sara still

was Sara!
Her life had clearly
been wing clipped.
Her job was gone
she couldn't drive
and she was imprisoned
in a treatment schedule.
Even her hair
had vanished.

Despite that
Sara was the same.
As we sat on the bench
under leafy trees
discussing everything
under the sun
I was relieved to see
how whole Sara was.
She lived and laughed
smiled and drank coffee.
Her voice was
strong and steady
her gaze and humor
sharp as always.

I had been afraid
to return to NJ
because I was sure
I would step into
a world of illness
like the final months
of my mother's life.
That I would
spend the summer
looking on helplessly
while yet another
beloved person
faded away.

But no.
This was OK.
Sara was
still Sara.
For now.

I had no idea
how long Sara
would remain
this healthy.
But seeing her
so full of life
was definitely
a gift.

While sun glittered
on the grass and
ducks swam by
on the long pond
the sorrow bird sat
in a nearby tree
and sang so quietly
I almost didn't hear.


Vickie wasn't with us
that morning in the park
but the next day
we talked on the phone
about Sara's condition
and treatment schedule.

During our conversation
I told Vickie something
that I had wanted to say
for a very long time.

I told her
'I'm in.'

By that I meant
I would stay with Sara
regardless of
how her cancer developed
regardless of
how long her illness went on
regardless of
how painful it became.

So it was
with my mother

and so it was now
with Sara.

I didn't say this to Sara.
But if I was a sorrow bird
I would have sung this song:
'Sara my Sara
I am here.
I can't heal you
but I can walk beside you
while you go through this.
I will not disappear
while you disappear.'

That summer
I met up with Sara
a few times a week.

Sometimes I also
accompanied her
to chemotherapy.

The first time I went
to Sara's treatment
Vickie drove us
to a hospital
near their home.
A sterile place
without warmth.

Because Sara was Sara
she brought the warmth.
She chatted with everyone
the receptionist
the nurses
the other patients.
Always with
the same smile
and sunny heart.

Sara wasn't naive
but she was outgoing
and naturally friendly
with an attitude that
lit up her surroundings.

That's what Sara
had done every day
in my mother's house
and that's what she did
in the depressing hospital.

As for me
I was anxious.
Never before
had I witnessed
someone's chemotherapy.

I followed Sara's lead and
was friendly with everyone.
But I loathed every second.
I hated that my friend
needed chemotherapy
and I hated that
she was a patient
and would remain one
until the day she died.

The treatment took
almost two hours.

The room was filled
with reclining chairs
without privacy screens.
Each patient was
surrounded by
beeping equipment
and other patients.

Sara sat with
a tube in her arm
and we talked
a little bit until
she closed her eyes
and fell asleep.

I went to the cafeteria
for a cup of coffee
lukewarm and weak.
As I walked the corridors
the sharp medicinal smell

permeating the air
made me nauseous.

Vickie was also there.
During the treatment
she kept an eye on Sara
talked to the personnel
asked a lot of questions
and essentially did
everything in her power
to make sure Sara
got what she needed.

Vickie reminded
me of me.
How I was with
my own mother
during doctor visits
medical treatments
and hospital stays.
She was learning
what I had to learn
namely how to be
my mother's advocate
in medicine's complex
and confusing world.

I knew how scared
Vickie was feeling
because I remembered
how scared I had been.

Now once again
I was frightened
although this time
for Sara's sake.

Vickie and I were joined
by our determination
not to lose our Sara.
No no no!
Not like this
attached to machines
in a depressing hospital
without soul.

One day Sara told me
that her treatment
was in jeopardy
due to a change
in her insurance.

Behind every single
treatment and pill
doctor visit and MRI
stood Sara's husband
and his benefits.
Frank held up
Sara's health care
through his job
which provided Sara
with medical insurance.
A huge pressure
he took care of
every single day.

Apart from the trouble
with her insurance
Sara and I rarely
talked about money.
One time she told me
chemotherapy treatments
cost about $17000 each
which thank goodness
was covered by insurance.

Once when I was
looking for something
in Sara's kitchen
I opened a drawer
jam-packed with
white envelopes.
A ghastly collection
of medical bills
MRI images
doctor's reports
insurance forms.

Cancer's paperwork.

I closed the drawer and
never opened it again.

The insurance problem
worked itself out.
Which meant Sara
now had a new doctor
at Sloan Kettering
the best cancer hospital
in the whole country.

As the Swedes say:
Good luck
in the middle
of bad luck.

There would be
no more journeys to
the depressing hospital.
Now Sara went to
a treatment center
in a posh area of NJ.
A modern building
surrounded by greenery
with high ceilings
calming colors and
homey furniture.

Despite the cozy decor
the ceiling corners
housed sturdy nests
built by sorrow birds.
All day every day
the air resonated with
their overlapping songs.

Going to Sloan Kettering
with my Sara
was not unlike
going to Starbucks
with my mother.

Everyone there
knew and liked Sara.

They appreciated her smile
and cheerful attitude.

Sometimes I was
alone with Sara
but most often
Sara's daughters
came along too.
And when Cirlei
Sara's glamorous sister
visited from Brazil
she joined us as well.

I wasn't the only one
who was determined
to stand beside Sara
during her journey.
We supported her and
we supported each other.
Proud members
of Team Sara.


First we found seats
on comfy sofas
on the ground floor.
We drank coffee
and ate snacks
until Sara was called
for her blood test.

The young man
who ran the tests
always smiled
when he saw Sara.
They had the same
sense of humor and
he was always kind
to our little gang.

After the blood test
we went up to
the second floor
and waited there
for Sara's treatment.
There was a big lounge

with free coffee
and more cushy sofas.

Sara was now avoiding
all dairy products
so I brought along
coconut milk
from Trader Joe's.
I fixed our coffee
and we sat in the lounge
with drinks and snacks
on the round wooden table
in front of our couches.

As we waited
we swapped stories
about the week just passed
or revisited memories
that made us laugh.
Almost always
we watched dog videos
on our phones.

We talked and joked
and we had fun.
Yes we did!
We were determined
to enjoy all the gifts
raining down on us
while Sara still
was Sara.

In the lounge
there were also
other patients.

Sometimes
it was difficult
to identify
who had cancer
and who had come
as support.

Many patients
still had hair

and could walk
by themselves.

Others were
more like Sara
without hair
maybe wearing a scarf
but otherwise healthy looking.

Some were extremely ill.
Slouched in wheelchairs
with hollowed-out eyes
and peculiar skin color
deep amber or chalk white.
Their withered bodies
clung to life by
the frailest of threads.

Those other patients
reminded me that
I needed to prepare
for the day when Sara
was in a wheelchair
while a healthier patient
sat nearby with friends
looking at dog videos
and drinking coffee
with coconut milk
from Trader Joe's.

Once two young men
handsome with dark hair
max 30 years old
sat on the other side
of the waiting room.
It was impossible
to determine
who was the patient.

Sara said to me
in a dampened voice
'When I see young people
sitting in this place
it's impossible for me
to feel sorry for myself.'

I understood.
No matter what
had happened to Sara
and no matter what
was about to happen
Sara had lived 56 years
on this earth.

That was also a gift.
One that was not
granted to everyone.

**A** nurse called out
Sara's name.

We all got up and
followed the nurse
to the treatment room
a large space with
screened-off areas
for each patient.
A private cubicle
that provided
a bit of dignity.

Each patient nook
had a reclining chair
for the patient and
a seat or two for
family and friends.
The personnel
almost always needed
to get more chairs
for Sara's gang.
Not that they minded.
They were surely
more upset when
a patient didn't have
any company at all.

The treatment started
with a nurse
asking questions
about Sara's health.
The nurse usually gave

a little advice
then stuck a needle
into Sara's arm.

The treatment took
30 minutes max.
Sometimes Sara lay
with her eyes shut.
Sometimes we chatted
about this and that.
According to Sara
the treatment itself
didn't hurt.

When it was over
we thanked the nurse
and went out exactly
as we had come in
with big smiles
and open hearts.

But you know what?
That's exactly what
we would have done
no matter where
we happened to be.
Sara always noticed
who was in the room
and always spoke with
as many people as possible.

Sara are you still talking?
Of course!
And why not?
While the trill of
the sorrow bird
grew in strength
Sara sang along
in the background
back straight
head held high.

That summer
Sara and I also
met at her house.

Sara's home sat
on a corner lot
with a grassy yard
on the left and
a concrete patio
in the back.

Sara's family lived
on the first floor and
in the finished basement
with tenants occupying
the second floor.

The first time
I went to Sara's house
that summer
she had arranged
a meeting for me
with Little Sarah and
their family friend Karla.
Sara had asked the girls
to teach me Instagram
so I could use it
to market my books.

That visit was also
when Sara gave me
keys to her house.

At that moment
with Sara so active
and full of life
it seemed impossible
to envision a day
when she couldn't
walk to the door
and let me in herself.

But we both knew
that day was coming
and when it did
we wanted to be sure
we were already ready.

My visits to Sara's house
followed a specific pattern.

When I put my key
in the building's front door
Lucky began to bark.
When I put my other key
in the door to Sara's home
and stepped inside
Lucky went berserk and
stood on his back legs
to get my attention.

Lucky needed proof
he had been seen
and he couldn't rest
until he was noticed.
A few kind words
and a pat on the head
always did the trick.

As soon as Lucky
had calmed down
I stood up and put
a bag of groceries
from Trader Joe's
on the counter.
Sara was only eating
organic produce
which Trader Joe's
had plenty of.
I lived next door
to Trader Joe's
so a little shopping
was an easy way
to help her out.

Next it was time
to walk Lucky.
If Sara and I
talked too long
Lucky got impatient
and started growling.
If we continued

he dug his nails
into my calves.

In the rigid hierarchy
of Lucky's dog world
I was beneath him and
always at his service.

I walked Lucky
because I loved
his eager company
and it was a way
to help Sara's family.
It was also a chance
to slip back into
the life I once had
with my mother.

By the way
when it was time
for me to leave
Lucky always forgot
we had taken a walk
two hours previously.

As soon as I picked up
my knapsack and keys
Lucky was beside me
barking eagerly
ready to go out
once again.

Of course we didn't
because I couldn't.
Whereupon Lucky
gave me a baffled look
his brown eyes
full of hurt.

Why won't you walk me?
Why aren't you staying?
Please don't go.

He didn't like it
when I disappeared.

Sara's home was
cozy and comfortable.

The kitchen and living room
were one large space
with a kitchen island
in the middle.

The home was crowded
but clean and orderly
with a tangible aura
of family warmth.

In Sara's house
you were never alone.
There was always
a daughter or two
maybe a husband
two dogs (one blind)
and various friends
who dropped by.

Guests were
always welcome.
Sit down!
Have some coffee!
How are you doing?

Just like my mother
Sara loved knickknacks.
She particularly liked
rearranging them and
setting out new ones.
Which meant her house
was a little different
each time I visited.

When Sara and I emptied
my mother's house
I had encouraged Sara
(and for that matter
everyone I talked to
for any reason at all)
to take what she wanted.
Which meant fragments
of my mother's life

popped up everywhere
in Sara's home.

A stone frog statue
a landscape painting
a porcelain Siamese cat
a blue-and-white teapot
two turquoise easy chairs
even my mother's perfume
L'Air Du Temps.

How nice to once again
find myself among
my mother's treasured things!
They made Sara's house
even cozier than
it already was.


When I came back
from walking Lucky
Sara had fixed coffee
with the electric kettle
and French press
that had previously
belonged to my mother.

We brought our coffee
over to the sofa.
The second we sat down
Lucky and Jordie
jumped up to join us.

As I mentioned
Sara wasn't interested
in talking about her illness.
Of course she updated me
on the latest developments.
We took care of that
at the start of my visits.

The most important news
was when Sara got results
from an MRI scan.
Brain cancer symptoms
can come and go

but only an MRI
tells the undiluted truth.

Strangely enough
the truth was not
always bad.
Once a tumor
actually shrank!

A joyful moment
and a tenuous oasis
in the perpetual storm.

As soon as Sara
had updated me
about her illness
we started talking
about all the things
we liked to talk about.

We talked about the future
the near future mostly
such as our plans
for the upcoming week.

We talked about the past
telling each other more
about our childhoods
and lives as young adults
including the pain
we still carried
from those years.

Our favorite topic
was my mother
and our four years
together with her.

Immersing ourselves
in shared memories
never got boring.
Our words were
a time capsule
flying us back
to a world where
our lives were whole

and the sorrow bird
sang instead of screeching.

**O**ne constant
during those visits
was the ringing
of Sara's cell phone.

Sara had a network
of family and friends
in NJ and Brazil
who called her regularly
at least a dozen people
maybe more.

They called not just
because Sara was ill
but rather because
they always called her.
It had been the same
when Sara worked
at my mother's house.

That cell phone.
I wondered
about it often.

When someone gets
diagnosed with cancer
it's natural and
maybe important
to ask the question:
Why did just this person
develop just this cancer?

As I mentioned
Sara liked to talk
on her cell phone
while she worked.
She squeezed the phone
between her ear
and her shoulder
in order to leave
her hands free.

I think Sara talked
while she worked
partly because
she wanted to connect
with people she loved
and partly because
it surely made
her tedious tasks
bearable.

Not that I ever heard
Sara complain
about her work.
But after many years
cleaning houses
Sara had bad knees
and maybe other issues
she never mentioned
at least not to me.

That cell phone.
I wondered
about it often.

Was it the cause
of Sara's cancer?
Maybe.
But Sara had grown up
on a tobacco farm
and living in the vicinity
of fresh tobacco
day in and day out
for many years
was surely not
particularly healthy.

I was curious
about the connection
between cell phones
and brain cancer
but I didn't google.
I honored my decision
not to dwell upon
the details of Sara's illness.

I knew
her diagnosis.
I knew
her prognosis.
I knew
that I was in.
End of discussion.

One day that summer
as we sat on the sofa
Sara took out her phone.

She showed me
the same pictures
Vickie had sent me
of the flawless spring day
when Sara was outside
for the first time in weeks
smiling in the park
surrounded by flowers.

As we looked at
the joyful pictures
Sara told me
'That was the day
I decided to stop
feeling sorry for myself.'

I nodded
too moved
to answer
or comment.

That statement was surely
the most courageous thing
I had ever heard anyone say.

It also gave me
a great deal
to think about.

I realized I felt
sorry for myself
because my best friend
had brain cancer
and I was forced

(I had chosen)
to watch her die.
Presumably slowly
and painfully.

I wish I could say
that summer day
when Sara and I
sat on the couch
looking at pictures
was the day
I finally stopped
feeling sorry for myself.

Maybe I did.
A little bit
in any case.

But one thing
I was sure of.
It was time
for me to stop
feeling sorry for Sara.
She didn't want that.
This was her life
it was her fate
and she wanted
to go through it
in her own way.

Sara my Sara.
I told you she held her head high.


That summer
Sara and I often went
out into the world.

Sara's white blood cells
kept increasing
and it became easier
to step outside and live.

Because Sara hadn't had
a seizure for six months
her doctor even said

she could drive again.
That was a happy day.

We did the things
we liked to do.
Walk Lucky
drink coffee
get pedicures
go out for lunch
visit thrift stores.

One day we went
to the Jersey Shore
with Sara's daughters.
We didn't swim but
strolled the promenade
alongside the beach.

The day was boiling hot.
I don't tolerate heat
and was close to fainting.
But still it was a delight
to watch Sara and
her beautiful daughters
walking under the blue sky
along the magnificent stretch
of glittering white sand.

That summer
Sara and I also did
practical things.

We took Lucky
to the vet
every other week
for a blood test.
A friendly office with
compassionate vets
and a kind receptionist.

The same thing
happened there
that happened
everywhere else.
We went in with

big smiles and
open hearts and
everyone loved Sara.

I admired the way
she freely discussed
her cancer with them
without looking for pity.

Sara also went
with Frank
to Ithaca NY
to take Little Sarah
to her second year
at Cornell University.
Wonderful that Sara
could still take part in
that classic parental ritual.

During our outings
Sara was happy
and always beautiful
in her little straw hat
or a stylish silk scarf
wrapped around her head.
Dressed in white pants
a flowered shirt
and her big smile.

That summer
there was an intensity
a shimmering urgency
in every moment
and in Sara herself.

One day we visited
my friend Jackie
who lived a few blocks
from Lucky's vet.
Later that evening
Jackie said to me
'Sara is glowing!'

I answered
'I know!'

Sara and I also planned
to go with Little Sarah
to the farmers market
located in Westfield
so Sara could buy
organic vegetables.

I knew that Michelle
my favorite yoga teacher
had a booth there
for her soap and candles
and other scented items.
After class one day
I told Michelle
I would be coming
to the farmer's market
with my friend
who had brain cancer
and wanted to buy
healing scents.

'Glioblastoma?'
Michelle asked.

'Yes' I answered.
'How did you know?'

Michelle told me that
a few years previously
she had lost
her best friend
to brain cancer.

After the diagnosis
Michelle's friend had
an operation and
Michelle visited her
at the hospital.

When Michelle arrived
she stood in front of
her friend's room
paralyzed by fear
unable to go in.

A nurse came
out of the room.
She saw Michelle
in the hallway
struggling.

Michelle told the nurse
'I just want my friend
to come back.'

The nurse pointed
toward the room
and said sternly
'That *is* your friend now
and she needs you!'

The story haunted me.
Would the day come
when I would be the one
hesitating outside
real or emotional rooms
and someone would need
to remind me sharply
'That *is* your friend now
and she needs you!'?

Michelle's story
was also a reminder
of our good luck
in the middle
of bad luck.
Michelle's friend
had changed forever
after her operation
whereas Sara
after her operation
was still Sara.
That was a gift.

At the farmers market
we visited Michelle's booth
and Sara herself
informed Michelle
that she had cancer.

Michelle was gracious
and kind as always
but surely it was
difficult for her
because she knew
Sara's future
Little Sarah's future
and mine too.

But just then
Sara was alive
and just then
she met Michelle.
That was when
Michelle became
part of Sara's life
and a deeper part
of mine.

Sara bought oils
scented candles
and skin lotion.
From then on
Michelle's products
permeated Sara's home
their soothing aromas
singing with love.

During that summer
Sara's poodle Jordie
had to be put to sleep.

A sad day for Sara
and her family.
But not for Lucky
who was now
the only dog
and at last had
the whole family's
undivided attention.

Vickie was the one
who took Jordie
to the vet and
stayed with him

as he died.
She was truly
a strong young woman.

Afterward the vet sent
a letter to the family
expressing his sympathy.
A fine gesture from
a good-hearted man.

Goodbye little Jordie.


There was one outing
Sara and I went on
which we kept secret
namely a visit to
a funeral home
to prearrange her burial.

Before my mother died
she did the same thing
at a funeral home
in Westfield.
I accompanied her
with gritted teeth
unwilling to embrace
the future pain
of my mother's
impending death.

To my surprise
the meeting was easy.
The funeral director
was friendly and
straightforward
as we went through
the practical details
of my mother's death.

At the end of our
hour-long meeting
we shook hands
and I admitted
to the director
that I felt relieved

because I had been
dreading our discussion.

The man nodded.
'This appointment
was the beginning
of your mourning.'

During that summer
I thought many times
that Sara really should
prearrange her funeral.
Particularly then
while Sara still
was Sara.

Before I figured out
how I could possibly
broach the subject
Sara told me herself
that she wanted to go.

We booked a time
and Sara asked me
not to tell anyone
especially her family.
She didn't want
to remind them
of the future.

The funeral home was
a cavernous building
in downtown Linden
with muted colors
hushed corridors
and ceiling corners
full of nests from
multiple sorrow birds.

Sara and I talked
with Beatrice
a sympathetic and
competent woman.

Sometimes
we spoke English

and sometimes
they spoke Spanish.
Sara and Beatrice
always apologized
when they needed
to change languages
but it was fine by me.
I wanted Sara
to feel comfortable
and to understand
all the details
about something
so very important.

Among other things
we discussed
urns
flowers
cremation
burial niches
organ donation.

The meeting lasted
almost an hour.
Details were ironed out
and papers were signed.

When we said goodbye
we had forged
a genuine bond
with Beatrice.
She felt like
a helpful friend
who would one day
help Sara's family.

Afterward we went
to Linden's city hall
and applied for
a parking sign
and disabled space
outside Sara's home.

The sign would
make it easier now

while Sara still
was able to drive.

It would also
make it easier later
for Sara's family
when they needed
to drive her.

Sara did everything
within her power
to help her family
before the day came
when she could no longer
help them herself.


**A**fter our errands
Sara drove us to
Rosedale Rosehill Cemetery
where she had just
purchased a niche
for her ashes.

According to the contract
with the funeral home
Sara did not yet have
a specific niche.
Instead her family
would choose one
after the cremation.

Sara and I decided
to look at the niches.
We drove to the middle
of the crowded cemetery
and parked in the silence.

Here and there
we saw freestanding
concrete walls
about five feet high
full of small niches
for the dead.

We went up close
to one of the walls.

Each niche bore
a bronze nameplate
and a bronze vase
to put flowers in.

Sara examined the wall
and its rows of niches.
It was a somber moment
so I waited for her
to break the silence.

'Perfect'
Sara said.
'My own little
studio apartment.'

We laughed.
Which is when
I learned that solemnity
is just one possible way
to handle something solemn.


As we stood by the niches
Sara told me that
this cemetery was famous
for one of its graves
namely a life-size
Mercedes-Benz
composed of granite.

A Chinese-American man
had promised to buy
his younger brother
a Mercedes-Benz
as soon as the boy
got his driver's license.
Tragically the boy
died at age 15
before he could get
the longed-for license.

Chinese custom says
that if you promise
something to someone
and the person dies

before you are able
to fulfill your promise
you must do your best
to keep your promise.
Which is why
the brother ordered
the granite Mercedes-Benz.

I said
'I need to see that.'

Sara said
'Let's find it.'

We drove through
the large graveyard
and after a while
found the car.
Life-size and made
of light gray stone
with impeccable details
including a license plate
bearing the nephew's name.

It might sound ridiculous
but it was touching
and really quite cool.

Sara sent pictures
to her daughters
not mentioning why
we happened to be
in the cemetery.

That day Sara and I
had a fantastic flow.
We checked off
two important errands
and in the bargain
found a Mercedes-Benz.

A melancholy flow
but still a flow
that humid afternoon
August 2019.

My fear
my dread
was the underscore
playing throughout
that fragile summer.

Whenever the sorrow bird
flapped its wings
the fluttering tips
scraped my heart.

I was afraid
of Sara's pain
because I didn't want
my friend to suffer.

My only comfort
was the thought
of morphine's power
which I had seen
up close during
my mother's last days.

I was also afraid
of how the tumors might
affect Sara's personality.

My only comfort
was the thought
of Michelle's story.
'That *is* your friend now
and she needs you!'
Regardless of
the coming changes
I was in and
would not disappear.

My biggest fear was
the emptiness afterward.
How would it feel
to live in a world
without Sara?

That was what
I found intolerable.

That was what
I could not bear.

That was what
I could not find
any comfort for
whatsoever.

As my mother had said
'I want Sara!'
That's what I wanted too.

Life without Sara!
If only I could
cover my ears and
block out that song!

But the chanting
of the sorrow bird
was like tinnitus.
Covering my ears
wouldn't help
because that dirge
came from within.

**D**espite everything
we still had hope.

Of course we did!
And why not?
Sara was still alive
and she was doing
everything she could
to keep herself well.
She attended her treatments
and took positive actions
to support her body
such as eating organic food
and drinking alkaline water.

Did those things help?
Maybe
maybe not.
But surely Sara
would have felt worse
if she had lost hope

and ate junk food
all day long.

It definitely helped Sara
to take constructive steps
and to have hope.
As the very wise
Portuguese proverb says:
Hope is the last to die.

Thank goodness for that!
You are alive
until you die
so what is the harm
of having hope?

The first time
that summer
when I told Sara
I didn't know
when I would
return to Sweden
she said firmly
'Don't stay here
because of me.
Go back like
you always do.'

I nodded
as if I agreed
although I didn't.

As summer went on
we discussed this
several times.
Finally I decided
to return to Sweden
in September and
stay my usual
three months.

It felt OK because
despite everything
Sara was OK.
The tumors hadn't grown

and one had even shrunk.
Sara barely had side effects
from her treatments
and she was even able
to drive her car.

Sara wanted me to go
because she wanted
both of us to live
our normal lives.
Of course
I wanted that too.

That was generous of Sara
because I would have stayed
if she had asked me to.


The week before
I left for Sweden
Sara told me
one of her legs
felt strange.
A bit numb.

The doctor said
it could be
a side effect
of the treatments.
Or possibly a sign
that the tumors
were growing.

All they could do
was wait until
Sara's next MRI.

We hoped
for the best
and prepared
for the worst.


My last visit to Sara
before I traveled

back to Sweden
was in the middle
of September.

It was still warm
not cool and frosty
like the Septembers
of my childhood.
Another world
in a different time.

As Sara and I sat
on her couch with
coffee cups in hand
and Lucky the dog
snuggled between us
Sara admitted that
she had been afraid
our summer together
would be sad.

'But' she said
'it wasn't sad at all.'

'I know' I agreed.
'We had so much fun.'

We sat quietly
for a moment.
I asked
one last time
'Are you sure
that it's OK
for me to leave?'

'Go' Sara said.
'It's time for you
to return to Sweden.'

# Autumn/Winter 2019

I stayed in Sweden from
the middle of September
to the middle of December.

Almost every day
I called Sara
not allowing
my cell phone
to touch my ear
instead holding it
at a safe distance.

Since I was
six hours ahead
I phoned Sara
late afternoon
my time
to reach her
in the morning
her time.

I called from different
parts of Stockholm.
Gamla Stan and City
Norrmalm and Vasastan
Östermalm and Södermalm
wherever I happened
to find myself and
whatever I happened
to be doing.
Anything from
sitting on a park bench
walking down a street
or drinking coffee
in the quiet back room
of a cozy café.

If I was home
at my hotel
I went outside
to Tegnérlunden
the small park
across the street

which actually had
better reception
for international calls.

I had a deep fondness
for Tegnérlunden
an odd little park
steep on all sides
and flat on top.

The park is famed
for a large statue
of the author
August Strindberg
but under a big tree
there's also a statue
of the author
Astrid Lindgren.
Just her head
and shoulders
with a book open
behind her like wings
and one of her characters
sitting on her shoulder
and a few children
nestled into her.

Tegnérlunden
also has a plaque
with a quote from
Astrid Lindgren's book
Mio My Mio
because Tegnérlunden
was where she saw
the melancholy boy
who was the seed
for that masterwork.

The first time I read
Mio My Mio
I saw that Astrid Lindgren
mentions my hotel's address
on the very first page.
I took a picture and

sent it proudly to
my Swedish friends.

Mio My Mio
is also where
she writes about
the sorrow bird.
The little boy hears
its plaintive song
throughout the story.

Astrid Lindgren
must have heard
the sorrow bird's song
when she saw
the sad little boy
alone on a bench
in Tegnérlunden.

I could hear it too
as I paced throughout
the little oasis of green
talking to my dying friend
as the afternoon light
slowly disappeared.

Sara and I usually
spoke for 15 minutes
sometimes longer
rarely shorter.

She always started
our conversations
the exact same way:
'Hello my dear!'

If there was something
important to share
concerning her health
Sara mentioned it
at the beginning.
Otherwise we discussed
everything under heaven
most often my mother
and our time with her.

It was however
impossible to avoid
Sara's illness.
Shortly after
I arrived in Sweden
Sara told me that
the numbness in her leg
and difficulty walking
were not side effects
of her treatments
but rather the result
of the tumors
which had grown
and now pressed
against a new part
of her brain.

The doctors wanted
to operate again.
They had a meeting
where they scrutinized
Sara's MRI images.
They concluded
that an operation
would simply be
too dangerous.

There was nothing
they could do
to help my Sara.
They only hoped
chemotherapy
might slow down
the course of the illness
and give her more time
hopefully quality time
without much suffering.

That was devastating news.

It was also distressing
to hear that Sara
was once again
having seizures

and once again was
forbidden to drive.

Unlike my mother
Sara accepted this.
Still it was sad
to hear that
a limitation
Sara thought
she had escaped
had returned.

Every setback
was an indication
that time was
running out.

To quote a sign
I once saw on a train:
The nearest exit
is behind you.

Despite the bad news
Sara still
was Sara.

Just as sharp
just as funny
just as warm
just as kind.

Sara was
still Sara.

I repeated
that incantation
many times
every day
to calm myself.

Sara was
still Sara.
And presumably
would remain so
until I once again
was back in NJ.

During every chat
I always told Sara
how many days
were left until
my return.

Occasionally I asked
if she wanted me
to come back earlier.
She always said
'No! Stay.
Have a good time
in Stockholm.'

Which I did
more or less
but still I missed
Sara terribly.

I held on tightly
to our daily calls
in a cold and dark city
that every day became
colder and darker.

Two times
Sara talked about
the future.

Once I mentioned Gast
my favorite café
in Stockholm.

Whereupon Sara said
'I'll visit you in Sweden
and we can go there
together.'

I closed my eyes.
If only she could!

A few days later
I said something
about Tegnérlunden.

Whereupon Sara
said again

'I'll visit you in Sweden
and we can go there
together.'

Again I closed my eyes.
If only she could!

Hope is truly
the last to die.

**I** had planned
to travel back to NJ
on December 16.

However
as my fingers hovered
over my keyboard
about to book
my two flights
I couldn't move.
As if something
was stopping me.

Such an odd sensation!
I tried to ignore it
but my gut said
I must absolutely
return to the US
at an earlier date.

I gave in and
chose a flight to NJ
December 10 2019
with a return flight
to Stockholm
March 12 2020.

That decision
that premonition
turned out to be
quite decisive.
Not about Sara
but actually something
altogether different.

We'll get back to that.

# Winter 2019-20

I landed in NJ
eager to meet Sara
but also a little nervous.

Before leaving Sweden
I had called Sara and
Vickie answered.

My whole body tensed.
Bad news was
surely on the way.

But it wasn't so awful.
Vickie said that Sara
wanted to warn me
she wasn't walking well
because her tumors
had gotten bigger.

'No problem' I said.
'Thanks so much
for letting me know.'

Nonetheless
the first time
I went to Sara's house
I had an enormous shock
that had nothing to do
with Sara's ability to walk.

Sara's face was
lumpy and crooked
and had swollen up
to at least twice
its normal size.
If I had seen her
out on the street
I probably wouldn't
have recognized her.

After greeting Lucky
and hugging Sara
I ran to the bathroom
where I sat on the toilet

and pressed my fingers
onto my eyelids
trying desperately
to hold back my tears.

After composing myself
I left the bathroom
put the leash on Lucky
and went outside.

As I walked
the happy little dog
I let my tears
flow freely.

When I came back
Sara was making coffee
standing at the counter
at a strange angle
her movements unsteady.

'Let me do it' I said.
'It's fun for me
to make coffee with
my mom's French press.'

I fixed our coffee
then sat beside Sara
on the couch
with Lucky the dog
nestled between us.

It was time
to get to know
and start to accept
this new Sara.

Because it wasn't
just Sara's face
that had changed.
Her speech was
slurry and slow
and she had gained
a lot of weight.

Sara's hair had
started to grow back

short and thick and gray.
That didn't seem odd
because I had also
stopped dying my hair.

But there was a place
on Sara's head
without any hair at all.
A shiny piece of skin
that I had never seen
or even known about
since Sara always wore
a flowery scarf or
little straw hat.

Later I found out
this was the place
where the surgeon
inserted a titanium plate
at the end of her surgery.

As for Sara's gait
it was slow
with one leg
dragging behind
but it wasn't as bad
as I had feared.

Despite all the changes
it was wonderful
to see each other.

Finally
I was back.

Finally
I was with my Sara.

This woman
*was* my friend now
and she needed me.

Later that evening
I did some googling
and learned that
Sara suffered from

something called
moon face.

A common side effect
of the steroids
she had to take
to shrink the swelling
inside her brain
that caused her seizures.

The steroids were
also the reason
Sara had gained
so much weight.

How was it possible
Sara had changed
so quickly?
I had only been away
77 days!

The sorrow bird
howled.


The shock over
Sara's transformation
gradually lessened.

With each passing day
I got used to Sara's
new face and new hair
new body and new gait.

But the changes
still made me sad.

That winter
a streaming site
started running
an ad about cancer.
A thin pale woman
without hair
in a hospital robe
stood by a window
and looked outside
longingly.

The picture changed
and now the woman
looked out through
the same window
rosy-cheeked
in normal clothes
long hair intact.

The ad alternated
between the images
in order to show
how it looks when
someone has cancer
and how it will look
when they get well.

I found that ad
unbearable.
O how I longed
to enter Sara's house
and be greeted by
the old Sara!
With long bronze hair
tight white jeans
happy and healthy
busy and bright.

Now I knew
what Michelle meant
when she told the nurse
'I just want my friend
to come back.'

Now I understood
the nurse's reply:
'That *is* your friend now
and she needs you!'

I had told Vickie
that I was in.
It was exactly this
that I needed
to be in for:
a Sara who

slowly was
no longer Sara.

A new song
with different lyrics
that sliced my ears
like razor blades.

**D**uring my 92 days
in NJ that winter
I didn't once go
to Sara's treatments.

Why not?
It wasn't something
we decided on.
The timing just never
seemed to work out.

Instead we met
at Sara's house.
The visits followed
our same pattern.
I entered the house
greeted Lucky
hugged Sara
walked Lucky
came back
drank coffee
on the couch.

Just like before
except now
I was the one
who made coffee
in the French press
while Sara waited
on the sofa.

We still talked
about the things
we always talked about.
Our conversations were
still gently interrupted
by Sara's family and friends.

Sara was
still Sara
talking and laughing
thinking and feeling.

But the truth
of Sara's illness
had become
more vivid
more palpable.

Not that Sara's home
ever felt depressing.
That never happened.
But the hope that wove
throughout the summer
was harder to find.
It wasn't gone altogether
but it had faded
into something pale.

It didn't help
that it was winter.
The days were not
as dark and cold
as in Stockholm
but it was still dark
and it was still cold.

I always left Sara's house
around three o'clock
at the edge of twilight
just before the sun
vanished completely.


It was almost impossible
for me to imagine
how it felt for Sara
to fade away
from herself.

I never devoted
much time to that.
It was too painful
to think about.

But once in a while
Sara did tell me
the many ways
her world had changed.

For example
how people acted
when they saw her
on the street
or in a store.
The recoil of fear!
The expression of shock!
What should they say?
What should they do?

As if it were unlucky
to be near Sara.
As if cancer
were infectious.
As if they were meeting
death itself.

Then there were others
who simply turned away
whenever they saw her.
As if by evading Sara
they could escape
the reality of death.

You couldn't blame them.
They didn't understand.
Perhaps they'd never
been close to someone
who had disappeared.

I was certainly
like that before
my mother's decline.
But once you experience
death at close range
it becomes a strand
in your DNA.

A ballad
whose words
you can't forget

because that song
from that sorrow bird
is set on repeat.

Despite everything
there were gifts.

One of the best was
when two people
who were part of
our common past
with my mother
re-entered our lives.

Megan
used to walk Lucky
and now she had
a grooming business
and visited Sara's house
every few weeks
with her white van
to wash and trim Lucky.

Lisa
one of my mother's
three masseuses
came every week
to massage Sara and
give her relief from
the pain in her leg.

Both women had been
friends of my mother
and quickly became
our friends too.

My mother
would have been
happy to see
Sara and Lucky and me
spending time with
Lisa and Megan
in a house full of
her favorite knickknacks.

She would have been pleased
that we had one another
even though we
no longer had her.

Sara and I
had both lost
so much
so quickly
and it was a balm
to get something back.


Christmastime.
Sara was staying
home with her family
so I decided to go
to Woodstock NY.

I booked a room
at KTD Monastery
where I used to study
Tibetan Buddhism.
Another world
in a different time.

In the days between
Christmas and New Year's
the monastery conducted
a special chanting practice.
The lingering scent
of Tibetan incense
floated throughout
the holy hallways.

I decided to ask
Khenpo Ugyen Tenzin
the monastery's abbot
to bless a Buddha statue
I had bought for Sara.

I spoke to one of
Khenpo's assistants
a kind woman
named Aileen

and gave her
the little buddha.

The next day I went
to Khenpo's rooms
and collected the statue.
A modest apartment
simple and clean
filled with Buddha statues
and other religious objects.

As a gesture of thanks
I gave him a card
with cash inside
as is customary
with such teachers
to help them avoid
handling cash.

A holy man
in a holy building
on a mountaintop
covered with snow
during the quiet week
after Christmas.
I felt I was in
the safest place
in the entire world.

Back in my room
I took the statue
out of its little bag
and held it gently
in my palm.

To my shock
the statue was warm
and pulsating.

I was dumbstruck
sure that my senses
were playing a trick.

The next day
I took the statue
out of the bag

once more.
Still warm
still pulsating.
As if the Buddha
had its own
miniature heart.

Back in NJ
I gave Sara
the little Buddha
and told her that
it had been blessed.
I took out my phone
and showed her a picture
of Khenpo Ugyen.

Sara was intrigued
and we made a plan
to visit the monastery
together in the summer.
(If only she could!)

Sara took the buddha
out of the bag.
She flinched.

'It's moving!'
she burst out.

I nodded.
'I know.'

Sara held the statue
against her cheek
and closed her eyes.

That winter
Sara and I met
outside of her home
only one time.

The occasion was
a potluck party
on a Sunday afternoon.
Sara's friends had
started these gatherings

a few months earlier.
Everyone wanted Sara
to get out of the house
and have some fun.
Everyone wanted
to spend time with Sara
while Sara still
was Sara.

I had already met
most of Sara's friends.
Paula and Sonia
Isabel and Rita
Paulina and Luisa.
They were all there
with their daughters.
All women.

The party took place
in a finished basement.
Sara had difficulty
walking from the car
into the house
and down the stairs.
No problem!
Sara's friends
surrounded her
and helped her take
every single step.

One room in the cellar
had a long table
overflowing with
Brazilian and
Portuguese food
including bacalhau
a delicious cod dish.
Another room had
a long table where
we could sit and eat.

Sara was radiant
stylishly dressed
in a gray sweater
and gray pillbox hat.

Whenever I happened
to glance around
I always saw her
talking
laughing
listening
quite simply
glowing.

The sorrow bird
was there of course
alone in a corner
quietly eating
a plate of bacalhau.

After a few hours
I was tired and hoarse
and ready to go home.
I looked for Sara
and saw she was
still talking
still shining.

If my mother had
been at the party
she would have teased
'Sara are you still talking?'

Yes mom she is!
Thank goodness.

I said goodbye
and left my Sara
in a good place
with warmhearted
family and friends
who loved her
just as much
as I loved her.

That afternoon
January 2020
there was a house
in a little NJ suburb
bursting at the seams

from all the love
blooming inside.

The next potluck
was already planned
for February.

Which meant
I would be able
to come along
one final time
before I traveled
back to Sweden.

As it turned out
the potluck I attended
was the very last
of those parties.

That January afternoon
as we ate and drank
talked and laughed
we had no idea
that party time
was almost over.

Not just for Sara
but for everyone
in the whole world.

It started slowly
with bad news
from a land far away.

An occasional drumbeat
about a novel virus
surfacing in China.

Certainly unfortunate
but definitely nothing
that would affect us
in the suburbs of NJ.

During the potluck
with Sara's friends
I had a conversation

with a young woman
about the new virus.

'Don't worry' I said.
'It's in China
so it's not going
to spread over here.'

Yep I was wrong
about that.

The drumbeat got
louder and louder
faster and faster
closer and closer.

The mysterious virus
marched resolutely from
one side of the world
over to the other.

By the end of February
people started using
the word pandemic.

But although corona
had begun to creep
into our vocabulary
it had not yet seeped
into our daily lives.

I still went to
Sara's house
yoga classes
12-step meetings
coffee with friends
in cafés and restaurants.

Some people got scared
and started canceling
upcoming trips
and other activities.

Sara's sister Cirlei
visited from Brazil
with her daughters.
Cirlei worked as

a travel agent and
she spent her days
pacing Sara's kitchen
talking on the phone
quickly and anxiously
in Portuguese.

Sara whispered to me
that Cirlei's clients were
canceling their trips.
Cirlei could only
look on helplessly as
her profession vanished.

Everyone was on edge
speculating about
what else in our lives
might be on the verge
of disappearing.

This was new territory
for all of us.
No one could predict
what was next.
All we could do
was wait and watch
while the drumbeat got
louder and louder
faster and faster
closer and closer.

Of course Sara and I
spoke about the virus.

We sat on the couch
with Lucky between us
drinking coffee and
following on TV
as corona continued
its relentless journey
across the globe.

We watched as
the virus emerged
in one country

after another.
We witnessed
the whole world
toppling like dominoes.

Despite everything
I never once thought
I wouldn't be able
to travel to Sweden.
Sara was OK
with me leaving
and that was what
my trip depended upon
not some virus
which no one I knew
had been infected by.

At least
not yet.

**W**e didn't understand
that our lifestyle was
teetering on collapse.

We didn't realize
that we only had
a few weeks left
until our routines
and reassuring habits
disappeared completely.

A before and an after
were on their way.
And what was before
would never come back.

# Spring 2020

On March 11
USA's president
(he who shall
not be named)
announced that
as of March 13
11.59 pm
Europeans could not
travel to the US.

He didn't say
Americans couldn't
travel to Europe
which was a relief
since I planned
to fly to Sweden
on March 12.

I left as scheduled
and landed in Sweden
Friday March 13.

A few days later
the EU announced
its own travel ban on
all inessential trips
(such as tourism)
to all EU countries
(such as Sweden)
by all non-citizens
(such as me).

Luckily I was
already in Sweden.
I had truly arrived
at the eleventh hour.

When I first heard
the EU's announcement
I recalled that strange feeling
when I was on the verge
of booking my flights.

If I had booked
my original dates
I would have been
stuck in the US.

The whole thing was
to say the least
extremely odd.

The world closed down.

Rock-solid borders
composed of rules
materialized overnight
between countries
and inside countries.
A new word rang out
all over the globe:
lockdown.

But not in Sweden.
Sweden went its own way.
Without lockdowns and
with recommendations
rather than restrictions.
Not even face masks
at least not then
at the pandemic's start.

The government advised
working from home and
avoiding public transportation.
To my amazement
the Swedish people
obeyed without protest.
The streets and subways
the squares and buses
were suddenly empty.
Stores and restaurants
shortened their hours
or closed down
altogether.

I visited
for example

my hairdresser.
The salon was open
but I was her only client
for the whole day
almost the whole week.

But overall
life in Stockholm
went on as normal.

I went to
the library
restaurants
bookstores
yoga classes
12-step meetings
cafés with friends.

Being in Sweden
felt like a rare piece
of good fortune
in a world swiftly
running out of luck.

I felt safe
and yes
I felt free.


The virus continued
its tenacious march
around the globe.

Travel was rapidly
becoming impossible
as ever more flights
got canceled.

The US government said
Americans abroad should
come home immediately
or be prepared to stay
wherever they were
for a very long time.

Swedish immigration said
if no flight was available

on your day of departure
non-citizens were allowed
to stay in Sweden
without being punished.
But you had to apply
for a visa extension
and not wait until
the very last minute.

I had always wanted
to live in Sweden
longer than my usual
90 tourist days.
This was my chance!
I couldn't leave
so I had to stay.

I sent my application
to immigration
and asked for
six extra months.
Surely by that time
the pandemic
would be over.

Yep I was wrong
about that as well.


As more countries
locked the door
behind themselves
it seemcd unlikely
I would be able
to return to the US.

It also became
more unlikely
internally.

By April 2020
NJ had become
the new epicenter.
Thousands were dying
every single week.

Being there was
truly dangerous.

Besides which
if I left Sweden
I had no idea
when I could
possibly come back.

The past seven years
I had spent at least
a third of my time
in Stockholm.
My heart and
yes my identity
were there and
I didn't want to be
anywhere else.

The thought of life
without Sweden
was intolerable.

**A**nd Sara?
Sara my Sara?

I decided not
to mention to her
that I might not be
coming back to NJ
in June as planned.

During our daily chat
I never said a word
about my application
to immigration.

But within my silence
a war was raging.

Just like the years
with my mother
I was caught in
a hellish tug-of-war:
Sara or me?
Duty or freedom?

On the one hand
Sara was not on
the verge of dying
despite the fact
that her condition
had gotten worse.
Some people with
glioblastoma
survive several years
even as long as five.
It felt like we
still had time.

On the other hand
I felt I was betraying
both Sara and myself.
How could I be in
when I found myself
3926 miles away
on the other side
of the Atlantic?

That woman
was my friend
and she needed me.

But wait!
I told myself.
This decision has
been made for you.
You can't go back
because you're stuck
in Sweden.

And yet I knew
I wasn't actually stuck.
Not really.

The American Embassy
in Stockholm
said it was possible
to fly to the US
from Frankfurt
if you really wanted to.

The problem was
I really didn't want to.
In a locked-down world
I found myself in
a rare free zone.
I wanted to stay
and not go back
to a social jail
reeking of death.

At the same time
I wanted to be with
my sick friend
my dying friend
who needed me.

The sorrow bird
was not happy
with my decision.
As I roamed about
springtime Stockholm
enjoying the city's
exquisite freedom
my ears burned
from the sorrow bird's
songs of dismay.

The days counted down
without an answer
from immigration.

As June came closer
it felt important
and ethical
to let Sara know
I would probably
be staying in Sweden.

The day I finally
decided to tell her
I stood with my phone
on Holländargatan
a side street close
to Tegnérlunden.

I hid in the shadows
of the stone buildings
and told Sara
I had applied for
a visa extension
and therefore
it was possible
I wouldn't be
returning in June
as planned.

Sara listened.
As soon as I had
stopped talking
she told me how
a friend of a friend
took three flights
in order to return to
the US from Portugal.

My heart cramped.
Sara was right.
If I really wanted
to come back
there was a way.

It would be expensive
it would be convoluted
it would take several days
but it was possible.

'We'll see' I said.
'I might not even
get the extension.'

I said that
even though
I was positive
I would get it.

Finally it was done.
Sara knew.

Duty or freedom?
I had chosen freedom.

The price I paid
was an inner shriek
a guilty reminder
that I had betrayed
my best friend.

Whenever I looked up
at the glorious spring sky
I saw a sorrow bird
perched on a rooftop
hanging its head
silent with shame.


Two weeks later
I got a letter
from immigration.
My application
for a visa extension
had been denied!

The letter said
that despite the lack
of direct flights from
Sweden to the US
there were other
available flights.
Therefore I needed
to take those flights
as soon as possible.

To my horror
the deadline
set by immigration
for my departure
had already passed.

The nearest exit
was behind me.

In a whirl of panic
I arranged my departure.
Sure enough
there were flights.
I found one from
Stockholm to London

and another from
London to New York.

Then I called Sara
and told her that
I would be back
in two days.
Which was actually
two weeks earlier
than originally planned.

The joy in her voice!
The delight and the glee!

In the middle of
all my confusion
Sara's happiness
was a priceless gift.


My friend Sheila
came to the hotel
to say goodbye.

While I frantically
packed up my room
I told Sheila
I felt humiliated by
immigration's rejection.

I also told Sheila
I didn't want
to leave my Swedish
bubble of freedom
and enter a locked-down
American world.

Besides which
I had no idea when
I could return to Sweden.
But if the travel ban
between US and Europe
was finally lifted
I could come back
in three months.

Sheila said
'For you
three months
means nothing
because you have
plenty of time.
But for Sara
three months
might just be
all the time
she has left.
I think this is good
and I'm sure that
one day soon
you'll come back
to Sweden.'

I stopped packing
and sat down.
Sheila was right.
For me
three months
was nothing.
For Sara
three months
just might
be everything.

That was the moment
I stopped feeling
sorry for myself.
That was the moment
I started preparing
to leave Swedish freedom
and unlock the door
to a closed country.
My country.

The sorrow bird
stretched its wings
and got ready for
its next journey.

Thanks Sheila.

At that point
in the pandemic
there were no
public covid tests
and no requirement
to show a negative test
in order to travel.

No tests were needed
since no one was traveling.
The world was still
in a state of shock.

You did however
need a face mask
in order to fly.
I went to stores
all over Stockholm
but no one sold masks
because no one wore them.

Finally I called
my friend Ylva
the only person I knew
who sometimes wore a mask.

Thank goodness Ylva
had a few to spare.
I rode an empty subway
over to her apartment
and got my very first mask.

Thanks Ylva.


The bus to the airport
was empty.

The airport itself
was deserted.

On the departures board
seven flights were listed
for the entire day.

The plane had at most
a dozen passengers.

I stretched out over
an entire row.

It felt like an unseen hand
had snapped its fingers
and made all the people
disappear like a dream.

It was scary
and surreal.
But inside
I felt clear.
In my heart
I was ready.

I knew what
I was leaving.
I knew where
I was going.

As Sweden receded
behind me
the US arose
ahead of me.

Farewell Stockholm!
I'll see you
when I see you.

# Summer 2020

I returned to NJ
Sunday May 24 2020.

I stepped into
a new world
a new reality
a new New Jersey.

In contrast to
life in Sweden
where there were
no masks for sale
everyone in NJ
wore a mask
and some people
even used two.

Trader Joe's had
an enormous sign
at the entrance
NO ADMISSION
WITHOUT A MASK!
IT'S THE LAW!

Yoga classes
were suspended.
12-step meetings
had disappeared.
My roommate Susannah
was stuck in Nicaragua
which meant I was
in her apartment
all by myself.

Stores and restaurants
had just opened again
but you weren't allowed
to go inside.

Supermarkets were open
but the number of shoppers
was severely limited
and you usually had

to stand outside
a very long time.

Everyone was frightened.
Everyone was paranoid.
Everyone was scared
of everyone else.

For me the worst thing
was when people learned
I had been in Sweden
and I watched them
back away from me
with terror in their eyes.

Sweden!
That shameless land
without lockdown!
The land that took
no responsibility
whatsoever!

That was the opinion
in the US just then.

After being away
for 73 days
I now was a stranger
in my native land
which was the only land
that would have me.


As soon as I was back
I spoke with Sara.
What a joy!

I also spoke with Vickie
who wondered
if I wouldn't mind
waiting 14 days
before visiting Sara
since her immune system
was so compromised.

I agreed.
Of course I agreed.

In that phase
of the pandemic
travelers were not
required to quarantine
because at that time
there were no travelers.
But anyway it felt
like a good idea.
The last thing
Sara needed
was covid.

There were also no
over-the-counter tests
available then
so there was no way
to confirm if
I was infected.

I just had to wait.

**V**ickie called me
the very next day
and said that Sara
wanted to see me.

'We can park the car
in front of your building
so you can talk with
my mom in the car
and you on the sidewalk.'

'Of course!'
I exclaimed.

'We're on our way'
she replied.

I went outside into
the burning-hot day
and waited impatiently
for Vickie's car.

When she pulled up
I ran toward them
tearful with euphoria.

Immediately
it became clear
that Sara was
in bad shape.

She still had
a moon face
and short hair
with a bald spot.
Plus she had gained
even more weight.

But now she was
oddly stiff.
Then I realized
Sara wasn't stiff.
She was paralyzed
unable to use
the arm and leg
on one side
of her body.

And it was more
than just that.
Something had
changed cognitively.
Sara's eyes were
wild and unfocused.
Her speech was
slow and thick
sometimes incoherent
almost childlike.

Was this the same woman
who I had talked with
every day in Stockholm?

I tried to hide my shock.
Apparently it didn't work
because Vickie said
'You didn't know
my mom was this bad.'

I looked at Sara.
She didn't react
to Vickie's words

but just kept staring
with a big smile
and wandering eyes.

Had Sara even understood
what Vickie had said?

'No' I answered.
'Definitely not.'

As I stood on the sidewalk
Sara and I chatted
about our daily lives
and the pandemic
which now was
our new daily life.

We made a plan
to talk every day
and then meet up
after my quarantine.

When we said goodbye
Sara and I couldn't hug
so we threw kisses.

I went into the apartment
and sat on my bed
shaken to the core.
How Sara must have
exerted herself during
our daily conversations
in order to sound
so happy and together!

Sara did that for me
because she didn't want me
to worry about her.

Sara did that for herself
because she wanted
to hold on to a life
that was slipping
out of her hands
at rapid speed.

I had a sudden urge
to fly back to Sweden
go to immigration and
thank them heartily
for rejecting me.

Then I would
turn around and
fly back to the US
and wait 14 days
until I could finally
be with my Sara.

That woman
*was* my friend now
and she needed me.

Thank goodness
I was back.


I had no idea why
Sara's condition
had deteriorated
so swiftly.

Tumors?
Seizures?
Medicine?

I got the answer
a few days later.

Still at home
in Sara-quarantine
unwilling to go out
into the heat and
wrestle with a world
that was scared of me
I was lying listlessly
on the leather sofa
when I got a call
from a sobbing Vickie.

The day before
she had spoken
with Sara's doctor

to get results from
the latest MRI.

The doctor said
the tumors had
grown substantially
and in her opinion
Sara had max
three months
left to live.

It felt as if an iron pipe
slammed into my heart.

My mind went silent.

Or maybe
it wasn't silence.
Maybe other noises
were drowned out
by the roaring thunder
of the sorrow bird's tears.


**V**ickie told me that
after they got the news
she drove Sara and
Little Sarah and Lucky
on an excursion to
a nearby waterfall.

That evening
Vickie sent pictures
from their day out.
Sara sat before
a spectacular waterfall
in her wheelchair
leaning awkwardly
over to one side.
She smiled and
made the peace sign
as well as she could
despite her paralysis
despite the horrible news.

Sara had lost
so much

but her spirit
was still intact.

I also understood
why they went
to the waterfall.
During an episode of
the Swedish TV series
Stars in the Castle
the comic Per Andersson
talked about how
he and his friends
handled the devastating loss
when their close friend
suddenly died young.

Per Andersson said
'Horrible things
happen in life.
That's just how it is.
But we were going
to try and push back.
We would give
life a fight.'

That little trip
to the waterfall
was a way for Sara
and her daughters
to push back and
give life a fight.

In the face of
horrendous news
they decided
not to go under
but instead experience
something splendid.

I told you they were brave.

Sara and I spoke
the next day.

She didn't mention
the doctor's news

so I decided not
to mention it either.

The days until
I could meet Sara
went slowly since
there was so little
I could actually do
due to the pandemic.

At the same time
the days until
I could meet Sara
went quickly since
she had so few
left to live.

The worst was that
despite our plan
to talk daily
we usually didn't.
Time and again
Vickie answered
Sara's cell phone
to say that Sara
didn't feel well
and couldn't talk.
Maybe try again
tomorrow.

But often tomorrow
didn't work either
which meant
many days passed
when I didn't hear
Sara's voice.

Sometimes
the sorrow bird
was mute.

One day during
my Sara-quarantine
I walked in the heat
to get an antibody test

because I was sure
I had gotten covid
in Sweden in March.

If I had antibodies
that meant I could
leave my quarantine
and go visit Sara
earlier than planned.

The test result
was negative.
I didn't have
a single antibody.

Perhaps I had
never had covid.
Or maybe
too much time
had elapsed since I did.

I was deeply disappointed
and didn't tell anyone
about the test.
Almost as if
I was ashamed
because I had failed.


**I** was alone
and I was lonely.

That sizzling-hot summer
I had so few ways
to distract myself
and so few friends
willing to meet with
someone who had
recently visited
dangerous
irresponsible
Sweden.

Despite my isolation
glimpses of light
occasionally appeared.

Due to the pandemic
my nephew Alexander
and my niece Flora
with her partner Henry
were now all in NJ.
That was a gift.

I visited Jackie
in Roselle Park.
A tremendous relief
to be with someone
kind and sympathetic.
She even gave me
a stylish face mask
with an image of
Hello Kitty.

I met Julia in
Mindowaskin Park
with cups of coffee
and face masks.

Merilyn and I met
at the Westfield Diner
which had moved
the whole restaurant
outdoors to the parking lot.

Several other friends
were also willing
to spend time with me.
I was grateful for
each and every one.

But mostly I was angry.
Angry at all the people
who were afraid of me.
Angry at the US
because it wasn't Sweden.
Angry at NJ's
militant strategy
of handling the virus.

I knew I needed
to be careful

and not express
such thoughts out loud.

Nevertheless one day
in the park with Julia
I shared with her
a toned-down version
of my bitter musings.

Julia listened carefully
then replied quietly
'You don't understand
what we went through.
You weren't here.'

It took time but
gradually I realized
Julia was right.
I wasn't there
when NY and NJ
were the epicenter
of the virus.

My friend Devon
for example
told me that when
she walked her dog
in Greenwich Village
they passed by
refrigerated trucks
filled to the brim
with frozen corpses
because the mortuaries
were unable to cope
with the thousands
of dead bodies.

That's what Devon did
while I was in Sweden
enjoying springtime.

I had been lucky
to be in Sweden
at the beginning
of the pandemic.
No doubt about that.

But now I was in NJ.
It was high time
to accept reality
and for god's sake
stop moaning and
put on a face mask.

**G**radually I adjusted
to the new reality.

I started carrying
several face masks
in my pocket and
I always put one on
whenever I went out
in downtown Westfield.

It was true I preferred
Sweden to the US
but at the end of the day
I was an American citizen.
When Sweden rejected me
the US welcomed me.

This was my country
despite everything.
A little gratitude was
definitely in order.

**A**fter Sara learned
she only had
three months left
she told her family
about our visit
to the funeral home.

Vickie called me
to talk about
the arrangements.
I was at home in
Sara-quarantine
lying on the sofa
in the living room
avoiding the heat.

I was alone
without Susannah
who was still trapped
in Nicaragua
and I was without
Rosie the cat
who had died
some months before.

I found the paperwork
then Vickie and I
discussed the details
of Sara's burial.
A conversation
neither of us wanted.

That girl!
Brave and courageous
mature and responsible
while she sorted out
the final threads
of her mother's life.

Just then
life demanded
something of Vickie
too heavy to carry
that nonetheless
had to be carried.

I understood
since life had asked
the same from me
a few years earlier.
That was a song
I knew by heart.

**W**hen quarantine
was almost over
I realized I had
no way to travel
to Sara's house.
I didn't have a car
and Uber's service
was suspended.

I asked a few friends
if they knew anyone
who I could pay
to drive me to Sara's.

Devon told me
her boyfriend Chris
like so many others
had lost his job.
He spent his days
fixing their house
in Cranford and
he had lots of time
to help me out.

Just like that
my problem
was solved.
A true gift.

Thanks Devon.


Finally the day came
when I could return
to Sara's home.

Lucky was still
affectionate and
lovably demanding.
Otherwise the house
was full of changes.

Both Sara's daughters
now lived at home.
Vickie was on leave
from work and
Little Sarah was back
from Cornell.
Frank was at work
despite the pandemic
which meant Sara
had health insurance
thank goodness.

A hospital bed
with a system of

harnesses and pulleys
sat in the middle
of the living room.
There was also
a steel wheelchair
waiting in the corner.

The biggest change
was my Sara.
Her paralysis meant
she could no longer
move by herself
sit up on her own
or feed herself.

The paralysis also made
swallowing difficult
so every meal
was full of peril.
It also meant Sara
had to wear a bib
and someone needed
to wipe off her face.

Because Sara was paralyzed
and on strong medication
she had difficulty reading
her own body signals.
After Sara had eaten
and several people had
exerted themselves
to move her from
the kitchen island
back to the hospital bed
Sara often called out
'I'm hungry!'

Her friends explained
she had just eaten.
Sometimes that worked
sometimes not.
If Sara persisted
there was nothing to do
but give her more food.

Vickie and Little Sarah
were the main caregivers
but they also had help
from Sara's friends.
The same women
I had talked to
and laughed with
at the potluck lunch
earlier that year.

Now everyone wore
resigned expressions
and inconsolable eyes
as they fed Sara
moved her
kept her clean
all the while
staying patient with
Sara's inability
to understand
her own body.

Sara our Sara.


**M**y self-chosen job
was caring for Lucky
mostly via long walks
which he needed and
enjoyed so much.

Sara loved Lucky
and I was sure
it warmed her heart
to see him happy.

As Lucky and I strolled
around the neighborhood
in the baking heat
I enjoyed his eager glee
and endless desire
to thoroughly smell
absolutely everything.

At the same time
during our walks

I steeled myself
for my return
to Sara's house
and the new Sara.

As I walked with
the lively little dog
a sorrow bird flew
just above my head
whispering repeatedly
'That woman
*is* your friend now
and she needs you!'

**A**fter walking Lucky
I made coffee
and sat beside Sara.

Our pattern had collapsed
but I fulfilled my part
as best I could.

I did it for Sara.
I did it for me.
I did it for Lucky.
I did it to help
Sara's family and friends.

Sometimes when
I returned with Lucky
Sara was still
being fed lunch
or fast asleep
in the hospital bed.

Once in a while
Sara and I were able
to have a short chat
and what a joy it was
to have genuine contact.

No matter what
Sara was doing
I always stayed
until three pm.

During all my visits
I wore a face mask.
One time Sara said
she wanted to see me
without the mask.
But it felt too dangerous.
The last thing I needed
was to bring covid
into that house and
cause more suffering
for my Sara.

The mask was also
for my sake.
If I got covid
I would possibly
be shut out from
Sara's final days
left on this earth.
I wanted to stay healthy
so we could be together
as much as possible.

And the sorrow bird?
Even with a mask
muffling its beak
its songs were
just as clear
just as crushing.


During that period
many things happened
in Sara's life which
I didn't know about
and maybe never will.

Even now I learn
new details about
those last months
mostly when her daughters
post pictures and thoughts
on social media.

I didn't know that
one night Sara tried

to get to the bathroom
all by herself.
She fell on the floor
where she lay for hours
without calling for help
because she didn't want
to wake up her family.

I didn't know that
Sara's doctor said
'If only you had
gotten a headache!
Maybe we could have
helped you sooner.'

Although those details
are painful to hear
I still want to know them.
They give me insight
into Sara's journey
a fuller picture of
her tremendous courage.

They also give me
an opportunity
to be a witness
even now
so long after
Sara's death.

There are moments
when all you can do
is be a witness.
But I believe
that's important too.
If someone sees
your suffering
you are not truly alone.

Sara my Sara.
I didn't want her
to feel alone.
Not then
and not now.

In the middle of
those last weeks
Lucky became ill
due to complications
with his diabetes.

Several times
in the middle of
the intolerable heat
Devon and Chris
drove Lucky and me
to the emergency vet.

Lucky got a bandage
with a little apparatus
to measure his blood sugar.
The round machine
was in a tight bandage
designed to prevent him
from taking it off.

Nonetheless
a few days later
the bandage was gone.
Clearly Lucky had
gnawed on it secretly.
I had to admire
his persistence.

During those afternoons
at the emergency vet
I couldn't be with Sara.
Although I was sorry
to lose any time
with my Sara
I knew Lucky's care
was essential for
Sara and her family.
They loved Lucky
just as much as
my mother and I did
when he lived with us.

It was a confusing time
for Lucky as well.

He knew life
in his household
had changed.
He realized Sara
wasn't well.
Maybe he sensed
he was once more
on the verge of losing
a beloved person.

This time however
Lucky didn't avoid Sara
like he had my mother
when she lay dying.

The opposite!
Lucky often hopped
up onto Sara's bed
and lay on top of her
his golden paws
neatly lined up
his head held high
like a sphinx or
guardian angel.

Sara was his person
and he was in.
Always.


Sara's last weeks
that burning-hot summer
were perhaps the loneliest
in my entire life.

May I never experience
such intense isolation
ever again.

Sara was dying
Lucky was sick
the pandemic raged
and I had no idea
when I could return
to my peaceful Sweden.

The heat was insufferable.
I shopped for food
and I went on walks
in the evenings when
the heat had abated.
But often I didn't
go out at all.

I was alone
in the apartment
without yoga
12-step meetings
or other activities
that helped me survive
my mother's last months.

It didn't help that
many people still
treated me like a leper
even though I had been
back from Sweden
for several weeks.
That made me furious
and even more isolated.

The worst was when
a 12-step friend
had a gathering at their house
and insisted everyone
come in their own car
presumably to avoid infection.

I had no car and
there was no Uber.
I desperately needed
my 12-step friends but
their rules shut me out.

I was in free fall.
The 12-step program
which had always
been there for me
didn't exist.

Although
that wasn't quite true.

All the meetings
had gone online but
I refused to participate.

Why?
Don't know.

Because I was spoiled
from my time in Sweden
where there were still
physical meetings?

Because it felt distasteful
to trust a screen
with private matters?

Because I was
quite simply
petulant?

Don't know.

When I ran into
people from 12-step
in downtown Westfield
I was cold and dismissive.
If I couldn't see them
the way we usually did
I didn't want
to see them at all.

A childish choice
lonely and unnecessary
and the only person
it hurt
was me.

I was angry at everyone
about everything
and it was often easiest
to be alone.

Then I got a gift.
A gift called Natthiko.

Björn Natthiko Lindeblad
a former forest monk

who after 17 years
of monastic life
in Thailand and elsewhere
took off his robes
returned to Sweden
and started a career
as a meditation teacher
and public speaker.

On June 26 2020
a Swedish radio show
aired a talk by Natthiko.
All of Sweden was
moved by his story
and I was too
as I listened from
my NJ suburb.

Natthiko spoke
about death.
His father's death
and his own
which was on its way
after his diagnosis with
the wasting disease ALS.

Most touching was
Natthiko's tribute
to his own body.
A body that gradually
was losing its ability
to walk and breathe
and read its own signals.

Despite the difficulties
Natthiko's body
kept on living
as best it could
and during his talk
a tearful Natthiko
thanked his body
for all its efforts.

(By the way
Natthiko was

a year younger
than Sara and me.)

I thought of Sara's body
which was also doing
the best it could
despite brain tumors
and strong medicine
not to mention paralysis.

I thought of my body
mostly my heart
and nervous system
which were also doing
the best they could
despite my despair
and isolation.

Poor bodies.

I discovered
a treasure trove of
Natthiko's teachings
on SoundCloud and
started listening to him
throughout the day.
Usually I fell asleep
to the sound of
his kind mellow voice.

With Natthiko
I found a friend
in the middle of
my screaming loneliness.

When I was almost deaf
from the sorrow bird's
strident wailing
I was still able
to hear Natthiko.

When I was unable to bear
anyone or anything
I could always bear
Natthiko.

Several months later
I wrote him an email
and thanked him for
saving me during
that wretched summer.

O Natthiko!
Now you're gone
and you are missed
by me and Sweden.
But your voice
wise and calm
lives on.

**M**y friends
were another gift.

They listened to me
and understood that
I needed them
to remember me
even I didn't
get in touch.
My silence
did not mean
I was OK.

I prayed to
Little Therese
my invisible friend
who had accompanied
both Sara and me
throughout this journey.

I texted Aileen
so she could tell
Khenpo Ugyen
that Sara only had
a few months left.
Aileen wrote back
that Khenpo Ugyen
wanted pictures
of Sara and me.
I sent them at once.

My cyber life
gave no clue
about the daily hell
I was living through.
It was a pretend world
where I could post
about my books and
have contact with
all the wonderful
readers and reviewers
who lived in my phone.

One day my friend Joan
wrote a message
under one of my posts
saying she was glad
things were going well
with my writing
but she would prefer
to hear more about
my personal life.

I messaged Joan
explaining about
Sara's illness.
I told her I needed
to keep social media
as an imaginary zone
without illness
without suffering
without the sorrow bird's
piercing howl.

The person who
people saw online
was not me.
The fictional Florence
helped me avoid
the bitter anguish
of the real Florence.

On the mirror in my room
I taped up a quote

from the book
As Bill Sees It:

Believe more deeply.
Hold your face
up to the Light
even though
for the moment
you do not see.


That summer
I continued working on
horror stories in Swedish.

After intensive editing
I arrived at the point
where it was time
to take a pause
from the text.

Taking breaks has
always been part of
my writing process.
But taking one then
as the pandemic raged
and Sara was dying
felt extremely unwise.

I was living
in an empty apartment
in an empty city
in an empty world.
Empty hands
would decimate me.

Suddenly I got
a flash of inspiration:
I could translate
the 13 stories
into English!

All right then.
Just like that I had
an enormous project
to devote myself to

and fill my days
for at least a year.

What a relief.
An incentive to get up
and a reason to go on.

I needed as many
as I could invent
because just then
I found myself
rather short of them.


Sometimes
the fog cleared
and Sara arose
to the surface
completely lucid.

She was still there
under the new body
the dying body.

Both the fog
and the clarity
could be painful
to witness.

A fog story:
One hot summer day
I went as always
to Sara's house.

As always I walked
Lucky the dog
and as always
I made coffee.

Cup in hand
I stood beside
the hospital bed
in the middle of
the living room.

Sara crooked a finger
and beckoned me
to come closer.

Her expression
was confused
as it often was
due to the pills
that eased the agony
of the many tumors
growing in her brain.

I took a step forward
and bent down to listen.

'There's a girl over there'
whispered Sara
gesturing nervously
toward the kitchen.
'She told me
she's my daughter.
Is it true?'

I looked over
and saw Little Sarah
standing in the corner
tapping on her phone.

A cold finger
touched my heart.

'That's true'
I whispered back.
'The girl is named Sarah.
She's the youngest
of your two daughters
and she loves you
very much.'

Sara nodded
and leaned back.
Her eyes became
a touch calmer.

'OK'
she whispered.
'OK.'

O Sara!
Sara my Sara.

**A** clarity story:

One hot summer day
I went as always
to Sara's house.

As always I walked
Lucky the dog
and as always
I made coffee.

Cup in hand
I sat on the edge
of Sara's bed and
asked how she felt.

Sara's eyes were
open and alert.
She looked at me
steadily and said
'A month ago
the doctor told me
I had three months left.
Which means that now
I only have two.'

Her eyes filled with tears.
During the many months
of her long illness
it was the first time
I saw that happen.

A desperate panic
rose up in me.
I took Sara's hand
and squeezed it softly.

In as calm a voice
as I could manage
I replied
'That's what they said
but let's see what
actually happens.'

'OK'
she nodded.
'OK.'

O Sara!
Sara my Sara.

**M**y beautiful friend.

That's what Elaine
called my mother
on her deathbed.
'Goodbye my beautiful friend.'

I began calling Sara that
when I came to her home.
'Hello my beautiful friend!'

Because Sara was beautiful.
Despite the moon face
despite the paralysis
despite the bald spot
despite the weight gain
despite her unfocused eyes
she was the most
beautiful best friend
I had ever known.

One day when
I visited Sara
and it was time
for me to go home
(this girl go home!)
Sara said to me
'Goodbye my beautiful friend.'

I hold that memory
close to my heart
as my most precious gift.

**A** light amid
those sad hot days
were my car trips with
Devon's boyfriend Chris
who drove me to Sara
three times a week.

Chris's presence
was like bookends

around my visits.
Always there
in the beginning.
Always there
in the end.

The drive between
Westfield and Linden
takes 25 minutes.
As music played
in the background
Chris and I talked about
the virus and politics
our dogs and travels abroad
dental work and favorite foods.
Both of us wore face masks
like two robbers in
an old Western film.

Those trips functioned
as a warm-up
and cool-down.
On the way
to seeing Sara
I was always
a little nervous
because I never knew
what I would find
when I stepped inside.

On the way home
from seeing Sara
my state of mind was
relieved if it went well
tender if it went poorly
with a sorrow that was
impossible to shake off.

Chris accepted me
regardless of my mood
and didn't care
if I didn't feel
like talking.

Chris was a gentle and
unassuming companion.
One of the few people
whose presence I could stand.
One of the few people
I wasn't angry at.

Despite the face masks
those drives were definitely
my most normal activity
during those months.
A short respite when
life felt like life
instead of a pale
skewed version
of itself.

Chris helped me practically.
He helped me emotionally.
He became a friend.
He was a gift.

Thanks Chris.


Sara rarely left home.
Even her doctor visits
took place online.

Which was just as well
considering how difficult
nay impossible
it had become for Sara
to walk or move at all.

But one day when
I came to the house
Sara's daughters said
'Our mom wants
a milkshake.
After you walk Lucky
we're going to drive
to an ice cream shop
and buy one for her.'

My heart melted.
The girls longed

to give their mother
something enjoyable
and not just let her
lie in a hospital bed
hour after hour
day after day
waiting for death.

It took 15 minutes
to use the harnesses
and move Sara
from the bed
to the wheelchair
then take her
out to the car.

The girls were accustomed
to moving their mother
and didn't need my help.
Instead I held Lucky
so he didn't run away
through the open door.

They finally got Sara
safely in the car
and that was when
Sara had a seizure.
Her stiff body shook
her eyes rolled backward
then she went limp.

The fear in the girls' eyes!
Their shaky voices
as they cried out
'Mom mom mom!'

That was the first time
I had ever seen
Sara have a seizure.
I stood on the sidewalk
frozen in fear.

The outing was
impossible now.
We needed to move
Sara back inside

but we were too scared
to lift her ourselves.

Vickie called her fiancé Jose
who lived around the corner.
Like many others
he now worked at home
and like many men
he had a covid beard.

The three of them lifted
Sara out of the car and
sat her in the wheelchair.
They rolled her
into the house
and moved her
onto the bed.

I stood on the sidelines
with Lucky in my arms
looking on helplessly.

Back in the hospital bed
Sara fell asleep at once
exhausted after her seizure.

I told the girls
to take a break
while I stayed with Sara.

And that's what I did.
I sat on the sofa
with a cup of coffee
and Lucky beside me
watching over
my beautiful friend
as she slept through
the warm afternoon.


**W**ednesday July 15
I went as always
to Sara's house.

Called out
'Hello my beautiful friend!'

walked the dog
made coffee.

Sara lay in the bed
in the living room.
She was awake and
surprisingly clear.

I sat down on
the edge of the bed
and we talked
like we used to.
A proper conversation
the longest we'd had
in a very long time.

As always
we talked about
old memories
that were happy
and other memories
not so happy
but important to discuss
since they were part
of our common history.

Sara and I also agreed
that although we wished
my mother was still alive
we were thankful
she hadn't been compelled
to experience the pandemic.

To be stuck inside
forbidden to go out
to Starbucks
her beauty treatments
or Rosie's Wine Bar
with her best friend Elaine
would have made my mother
depressed and apathetic.

Not to mention face masks!
My mother definitely
would have hated them
not least because a mask

would mess up her hair.
That would have been
yet another reason
for me to be bossy
and her to be stubborn.

In my heart
I was also thankful
my mother wasn't alive
to live through Sara's illness.
That would have destroyed
my mother completely.

I kept that thought
to myself.

That afternoon
was a golden moment
an oasis of time
when Sara
once again
became Sara
and she and I
once again
had a chance to do
what we liked best.

That was a gift.


Friday July 17.
Two days later.

When I walked
into Sara's house
she lay in bed
completely silent.

When I said
'Hello my beautiful friend!'
she didn't look at me.

Vickie told me
Sara wouldn't eat
or get out of bed.
She had horrible pain
and was on morphine.

Three years before
Sara and I had given
morphine to my mother.
Now Sara was the one
getting morphine.
Time had gone so fast!

I walked Lucky
made coffee
sat on the edge
of the hospital bed.

Sara's eyes opened.
'You're here'
she said weakly.

'Of course' I said.
'How's it going?'

Sara had to swallow
before she could speak.
'I never thought
it was possible to get
a migraine in my eye
but now I have one.'

I said 'I'm so sorry.'

With sudden energy
Sara shook her head
vigorously and
waved her hands
dismissively.

'No!' she said.
'Don't be like that!'

'OK'
I said in surprise.
'OK.'

It took a moment
for me to realize
what had happened.

When I said
'I'm so sorry'
I meant

'I'm sorry that
you feel like this.'

Sara however
thought I meant
'I feel sorry for you.'

Sara was in incredible pain
and could hardly move
but nonetheless she used
the tiny bit of strength
she still had left
to make it very clear
she didn't want me
to feel sorry for her.

I told you she was beautiful.


I took Sara's hand.
She held it hard
and closed her eyes.

In the 1970 film
Love Story
a young couple
fall in love
and soon after
the girl gets cancer.

In one of the final scenes
she is dying and
her boyfriend comes
to the hospital.
It's nighttime and
the room is dark.
She is lying in bed
connected to machines
by a series of tubes.

Despite the equipment
her boyfriend gets
into the bed
and holds her.
They lie together
in the dark
in silence.

I saw that film
once as a teenager
but I never forgot
that scene.

So it was now.
I held Sara's hand
but I longed
to lay beside her
hug her and say
'I am here.
I cannot fix
this for you
but I am here
and I love you.'

No I didn't get
into Sara's bed
but I took her hand
and held it in mine.

We sat like that
all afternoon
in silence.

At five minutes to three
it was almost time
for Chris to come
and drive me home.

Almost time
to say goodbye
to my beautiful friend.

Sara was still asleep.
I didn't want
to wake her
but I needed
to loosen my hand
from our laced fingers.

One by one
I lifted her fingers
and freed my hand.

One finger
then another
then one more
then the last.

I drew my thumb
out of her palm
and whispered
'See you on Monday
my beautiful friend.'

Sunday July 19
two days later.

I woke up
just after eight.

I checked my phone.
The display said
Vickie had called
at 7.38 am.

I knew right away
that Sara was gone.

After my mother died
it took several months
before I understood
she truly was gone.

I knew she was dead.
Of course I did!
I had been there
when it happened.

It was rather that
in the months
after her death
I was so busy with
my mother's life
her house and garden
friends and money
insurance and taxes
and leaking oil tank.
How was it possible

my mother was gone
when she still had
so many things
to take care of?

December 2017
seven months after
my mother's death
I went to Berget
a retreat center
located in Dalarna
in central Sweden.
I craved silence and
my friend Monica
recommended Berget
as a place to go
and simply be quiet.

By chance
my weekend there
started just after
the new owners of
my mother's house
received the keys.
Our keys.

By chance
Berget was holding
a silent retreat
during my weekend
which meant I was
encircled by silence.
To enter the mood
I decided to
also stay mute.

An elderly nun
who lived there
kept an eye on me.
When I saw her
in the hushed corridors
she nodded at me
silently asking
'Are you OK?'

I nodded back
silently answering
'I'm OK
more or less.'

I did little that weekend.
Drank too much
strong Swedish coffee.
Read a book
from the library
about mourning.
Took soothing walks
in pine forests
filled with deep snow.

One afternoon
I returned to my room
after walking in the forest.
The little room glowed
with winter sunlight
a shimmering dance
of delicate gold particles.

I sat on my bed.
And that was when
a voice in my head
a voice in my heart
said ever so gently
'She's gone.'

That was the moment
the truth of her death
finally landed.

That was the moment
I stopped running
and finally accepted it.

The sorrow bird
had been waiting
for me to put down
my responsibilities
so it could whisper
as softly as possible
the cheerless truth

that my mother
was gone.

Sitting amid
the golden glow
of winter light
I wept a long time.

Afterward I felt
a clean peace.
All those months
I had used up
so much energy
holding the truth
at arm's length.

It was a physical relief
to stop fighting a battle
I could never win.

Yes I was still
emotionally fragile
but now my heart
was firmly anchored
in the truth.

With Sara
it was different.

As soon as I saw
Vickie had called
unusually early
I felt the truth
in every bone.

She's gone.

What am I supposed to do
without you?

How am I supposed to go on
without you?

How am I supposed to live
on this earth
without you?

# Part 3

# Without Sara

# 2020–22

# Late Summer 2020

Ice cream
was a food
I ate compulsively
during the years
my eating disorder
was at its worst.

Nowadays
I eat it seldom
a few times a year
at most.

The morning
I got the news
about Sara's death
I threw on my clothes
rushed to Stop & Shop
and bought a carton
of my favorite ice cream
Ben & Jerry's
Coffee Heath Bar Crunch.

Back in my room
I ate the whole carton
in one sitting.

Which is not
as self-destructive
as it might sound.

I know this because
one evening
after my mother died
I was alone in the
half-empty house.
It was shortly after
Lucky and Mooch
had moved away to
their new homes and
I missed them terribly.

My friend Maribeth
called and asked
how I was doing.

Instead of pretending
I was engaged in
something sensible
I told her the truth.
'I'm lying on the sofa
eating red velvet cupcakes
and watching Sex and the City.'

'Excellent!' she said.
'That sounds like
good grieving.'

I laughed
although Maribeth
wasn't joking.

I liked the idea
of good grieving.
That's probably why
when Sara died
I treated myself
to something that
made me happy.

A poor choice
for the body
but an excellent choice
for the soul.


The day vibrated with
a strange fragility
a quivering emptiness.

I stayed inside.
Partly because
it was too warm
to go outside.
Partly because
Westfield was
mostly closed
due to corona.

After eating ice cream
I did my writing
had a Swedish lesson
listened to Natthiko.

I definitely didn't
take a shower.

I wrote an email
to KTD Monastery
and ordered a lamp
in Sara's memory.
The lamp would
stay lit for 49 days
because Tibetan Buddhists
believe that's how long
it takes for humans
to reincarnate.

I sent Aileen a text
to share the news with
her and Khenpo Ugyen.
I called my sponsor Joanna
and wrote emails to friends
who had walked beside me
throughout Sara's journey.

The sorrow bird
roosted on my shoulder
all day long.
It leaned its head
against mine
and dug its talons
into my flesh.
It sang a song
woven of weeping.

The day was not
without surprises.
And gifts.

My sponsor Joanna
called to tell me
about an outdoor
12-step meeting
that evening in
Mindowaskin Park
a three-minute walk
from where I lived.

A meeting
right in Westfield!
A meeting
I could walk to!

58 long days
had passed since
my last meeting.
Usually I went daily
and the lack of meetings
surely contributed to
my emotional imbalance.

The meeting
began at 6.30 pm.
Although it was evening
the air was blistering
like every day
that sad summer.

Unfortunately
the meeting
was not normal.
The person in charge
had good intentions
but a dozen alcoholics
in a sizzling-hot park
sitting six feet apart
wearing face masks
was truly a recipe
for chaos.

We struggled
to hear one another
and most people
talked too long
desperate to shake off
months of isolation.
Clearly I wasn't
the only person
drowning in loneliness.

Despite the difficulties
the meeting was
a balm for the soul.

People read aloud
from the familiar
and comforting texts.
When my turn
came to share
I talked about
losing my Sara.

I left early.
The park was too warm
the meeting too messy
and I was too broken.

But exactly like
the yoga class
in the dark of Svalbard
the meeting in the park
lit a tiny inner light.

I couldn't get
everything I needed
but I got a little and
that was enough
to go forward.

In any case
forward to
the next breath.


After the meeting
I lay in bed
watching a film
when I got a text
from Aileen.

She told me that
Khenpo Ugyen
had just interrupted
the Medicine Buddha
chanting ceremony
and asked everyone
to switch over to
the Amitabha Buddha
chanting ceremony
dedicated to Sara.

Aileen told me
to go on Facebook
where the chanting
was streaming live.
I did so at once.

The ceremony took place
in the shrine room.
A golden space with
a huge Buddha statue
and monks sitting
cross-legged on cushions
chanting in Tibetan
behind long low tables
bearing their texts.

That room
was so familiar.
I had sat there
countless times
over many years.
Another world
in a different time.

I had contacted Aileen
in the hope that
Khenpo Ugyen
would include Sara
in his prayers.

I never expected
an entire ceremony
dedicated to my Sara
to help her make
the transition to
her next life.

I don't know
if people reincarnate
but if they do
Sara was not just
in good hands
but rather in
the very best.

The ceremony
lasted 30 minutes.
I didn't understand
a single word
but I listened
to the very end.

I didn't know that
the sorrow bird
spoke Tibetan.
But the sorrow bird
was full of surprises
and now and then
a gift.

Friday July 23 at 11 am
four days after Sara's death
her ashes were to be placed
in an outdoor niche in
Rosedale Rosehill Cemetery.

There would not be
a reception afterward
since gatherings
were forbidden
due to covid.

Chris drove me
to Sara's house
and refused to take
his usual payment.
A truly gracious gesture.

I came early
to walk Lucky
for the last time.
Saying goodbye
to my dog-brother
made a heavy day
even heavier.

Back at Sara's house
I made coffee
and sat down

on the couch
with Lucky.

The hospital bed
was gone.

I talked with
Frank and Vickie
and Little Sarah
about Sara's mass
due to take place
two days later.

I saw the mass cards
with Sara's picture
on one side and
the St. Francis Prayer
on the other.

There was also
a poster-size
photo of Sara
intended to stand
in front of the altar
during the mass.

The picture was from
that day in the park
the previous spring
when Sara decided
she would no longer
feel sorry for herself.

When I saw the photo
I told the others
what Sara had told me
about that day
and that image.

Frank's head jerked back
and his eyes sparked.

Sara's courage
once again
lit up the room
despite the fact
she was gone.

But as it turned out
Sara wasn't gone.
Not entirely.

I hadn't noticed
a little box sitting
on the kitchen island.
But when we got up
to leave for the service
Frank picked up
the small box
and said warmly
'Come on mami.'

Which is when
I understood
it was my Sara
in that box.

Her ashes
in any case.


In addition to
the usual heat and
unbearable humidity
the sky was filled with
angry black clouds.

A ferocious rainstorm
loomed in the air
ready to erupt
at any moment.

Sure enough
just as we pulled
into the parking lot
of the cemetery
the sky exploded.

What rain!
Not a gentle shower
one could run through
and get a little damp.
This skyfall was
a biblical torrent

a violent waterfall
a chaotic deluge.

The rain left
all the mourners
paralyzed with
nothing to do but
wait in their vehicles.

As the rain lashed
the roof of our car
I sat quietly
with Sara's family
and the little box
containing her ashes.

The time when
the ceremony
should have started
came and went.

We remained mute
listening mournfully
as the rain pummeled
the roof of the car
like machine-gun fire.

Vickie looked out
the car window and
broke the silence
declaring wistfully
'Mom always said
she would be late
to her own funeral.
Now she's done it.'

Gradually
little by little
the rain lessened
then stopped.

The clouds remained
heavy and gray
still hovering on
the verge of bursting.

The waiting cars
drove together
into the cemetery
and parked beside
the outdoor wall
where Sara's family
had chosen her niche.

Sara would have been
delighted to see
that her niche was
within eyesight of
the granite Mercedes-Benz.

Around 30 people
stood by the wall.

The priest started
the graveside service
but I didn't hear
a single word
and that's because
I started to rain.

A cry detonated
from the depth
of my stomach.
My sobs were
so convulsive
I could feel them
deep in my guts.

Life felt
only bleak.
Absolutely
intolerable.

The same thing
had happened
when my sister Diane
died November 2010.
For days on end
I could hardly breathe
because my stomach
had tightened into
a hard ball of pain.

I broke through
my emotional impasse
by promising myself
not to be destroyed
by Diane's death.
Instead I would
let my sorrow
teach me something
and turn me into
a better person.

But as I stood
by Sara's niche
I was too weak
to make promises.

I had swallowed
a sorrow bird
and all I could do
was drown.

That was when
Karla came over
and hugged me.

She surely sensed
I was hurtling
toward the abyss.

Karla said
'If you need
anything at all
just call us.'

Her words
were a buoy
of kindness.
A hand to
hold on to
in the eye
of my storm.

Karla pulled me up
out of the darkness.
Just a little
but a little

was all I needed
to go forward.

In any case
forward to
the next breath.

Thanks Karla.

**O**n the way back
to Sara's house
in the car with
Vickie and Frank
and Little Sarah
I suddenly felt
very strongly
that I loved them.

I longed to
say it aloud
but I felt shy.

Then I thought
Don't think that.
It's OK to say it.

I opened my mouth
and the words flew out.
'I love you.'

All three of them
turned their heads
and looked at me.

As if it was
the simplest
most natural thing
in the entire world
Vickie replied
'We love you too.'

**O**ne more thing
about that day.

Vickie had told me
that in addition to

the urn containing
my Sara's ashes
the niche had room
for other small items
to be placed inside.

Sara asked for
her cell phone
to be buried with her
since it had been
her connection to
family and friends
over the whole world.

Back in Westfield
after the burial
lying on my bed
numb and alone
I got an idea
for a short story.

A woman dies
and is buried
in a niche
with her phone.
Afterward
her best friend
calls the phone
to once again hear
her dead friend's voice
on the voicemail greeting.

The best friend
makes the call
but instead of voicemail
the phone is answered
by her dead friend!

The best friend finds
a way to shrink herself
and get into the niche.
She discovers that
the niche is actually
a studio apartment
cozy and charming

where a tiny version
of her deceased friend
is alive and well.

The best friend decides
to stay in the niche
and leave the world
permanently.

A good idea
for a short story
but I realized
I mustn't write it.

Instinctively I knew
that the story was
deeply unsound
and did not bode well
for my mental health.

It reminded me
of the classic line
from the film
Withnail and I:
We are indeed drifting into
the arena of the unwell.

There and then
I dropped the idea.
(If there is anyone
who wants to use it
please be my guest.)

During that black day
I could hardly form
a whole sentence
but at least I knew
it was a bad idea
to imagine myself
moving in with Sara.
That fantasy world
was a dark space
and if I went inside
I might never
find my way out.

I also decided
it was a bad idea
to visit Sara's niche
in the future.
It triggered something
unhealthy in me
a perilous whispering
from a deranged and
desperate sorrow bird.

The day after Sara's burial
I ran into Little Sarah
outside of Trader Joe's.

She was wearing a sundress
and holding a bouquet
of blue and white flowers.

We chatted briefly
and I asked her what
she was doing that day.

She replied
'I'm on my way
to visit my mom.'

Her words
her bearing
her flowers
felt innocent
and uncomplicated.

Little Sarah was
going to visit.
She had no plans
to move in.

I yearned for
a role model
to show me how
to grieve sensibly
not darkly.
Which is when life
sent me Little Sarah

and her bouquet of
blue and white flowers.

Thanks Little Sarah.


Sunday July 26 at 9 am
five days after Sara's death
her mass was held at
Immaculate Heart
of Mary Church
in Newark NJ.

I went with Lisa
one of my mother's
three masseuses
also Sara's masseuse
as well as my friend.

Everyone wore masks
and sat at a distance
from everyone else.
A mass without
physical contact
between mourners
was a woeful experience.
As if we weren't
sad enough already.

Frank and Vickie
and Little Sarah
sat close together
in the first row.
How odd it was
to see those three
without Sara.

Next to the altar
stood the poster
of Sara in the park
among the flowers
her head wrapped
in a colorful scarf
wearing big sunglasses
and a radiant smile.
The day Sara decided

she would no longer
feel sorry for herself.

The mass was short.
Afterward we stood
outside the church
on the sidewalk.
The ban on hugging
was still in force
and we did not
touch one another.

That day was also
much too warm
but since it was
not yet 10 am
the heat was bearable.

But only just.

After Sara died
I had no reason
to stay in NJ.

Especially then
in the early months
of the pandemic.
A world without
yoga classes
12-step meetings
normal socializing.

Every day
felt the same.
Like being trapped
in a fish bowl
limited within
invisible walls
endlessly repeating
the same empty pattern.

I listened daily
to Swedish news
eager for any signs
of Sweden reopening
to American tourists.

Alas the border was
still closed tight with
no change in sight.

I started thinking
about London.
When corona came
Great Britain never
closed its borders to
their cousins overseas
due to our countries'
special relationship.

I didn't know
a soul in London
but I knew the city
had Swedish expats.
Surely I could find
a few Swedes and
practice the language
which felt impossible
in little Westfield.

One day in June
I heard on Swedish news
that hotels in the UK
would reopen July 4.
The reportage included
a soundbite of cheers
from England's parliament.

Sara was alive then
but I saved those cheers
in my back pocket
because I knew that
if (when) Sara died
I just might need them.


Sure enough
when Sara died
I knew it was time
to go to London.

Part of me wanted
to drive to the airport
right after Sara's mass.

But no.
I could barely manage
to leave the apartment
and buy a loaf of bread.
I certainly wasn't
strong enough yet
for such a long trip.

I also wasn't ready
to leave Sara
and her daughters.

I decided to stay
in Westfield
six more weeks
then fly to London
September 1.

I would stay abroad
and I would not
come back.


During my final
six weeks in NJ
I clung tightly to
my daily routine.

My mornings
were devoted
to short stories
and Swedish lessons.
Otherwise I read books
listened to Natthiko
watched Swedish series
walked in the evenings.

I took actions
and I functioned
but I was broken.

I wandered around
with hollow hands
and a paralyzed heart.

A mute weight
had lodged itself
deep in my throat.
It refused to come up
and would not go down.

I was also sensitive.
Far too sensitive.
My nerves flamed
like a sunburn
beneath my skin.

My friend Senjin
who had died
many years before
once said sadness
could be beautiful.

I knew this was true
because I had felt
that kind of sadness
previously in my life.

This sadness however
was not beautiful.
A sorrow bird waited
around every corner
and lunged at me
with its sharp beak
pecking ruthlessly
at my shattered heart.

The air around me
was permeated
with sorrow.

I smelt of sorrow.

The perpetual sauna
of hot humid weather
intensified my distress.
It was difficult
to breathe properly

and taking a walk
through the thick air
felt like punishment.

There was nothing
I truly enjoyed.
I stayed in my room
with its steady stream
of air-conditioning
and made time pass
as best I could
waiting for the day
when I could fly
away to London.

Susannah was finally
allowed to leave Nicaragua
and return to NJ.

That was a relief.
Now I was no longer
alone in the apartment.

I had other friends
to hang out with
who didn't mind
my mourning.

But I still refused
to attend online
12-step meetings.
That was probably
my biggest mistake
that dismal summer.

My yoga studio started
holding classes outside.
But they took place in
the middle of the day
in the stifling heat
so I never went.

One evening they had
a restorative yoga class.
I went and saw
people I knew.

But I couldn't bear
pandemic small talk
so I set my mat
in a far corner
beside a sorrow bird
and stretched silently.

Camilla Grebe's book
The Ice Beneath Her
opens with an Inuit proverb:
You do not know
who is your friend
or who is your enemy
until the ice beneath you
starts to break.

It wasn't just Sara
who I lost that summer.
When I told my friends
Sara only had
three months left
most of them were
deeply compassionate
and stayed by my side
even if they lived far away.

But some friends
simply vanished.

When they finally
got in touch
it was months
after Sara's death.
Much too late
to hear them ask
'How are you?
How is Sara?'

I dislike conflict
but nonetheless
I confronted those
who had disappeared.

I heard excuses
which I judged

to be flimsy.
When I was young
I was the queen
of flimsy excuses.
But no longer.
A sorrow bird was
stuck in my throat
and the only thing
I could swallow
was the truth.

I got angry and
it was difficult
to forgive them.

With one friend
we sorted it out
immediately.

With two others
it took time
but we did heal
thank goodness.

But with another friend
an American friend
things still feel broken.

I think I know
what happened
with those friends.
The sorrow bird
scared them away.
Is there anything
more disturbing
than someone with
a shrieking bird
jammed in their throat?

I think I also know
what happened with me
and why my friends'
silence and absence
felt like a betrayal.

If someone ignored
the sorrow bird
they also ignored
my Sara.
And if I couldn't
discuss Sara
she didn't exist.
As if she were dying
all over again.

That summer I learned
there are many ways
people can disappear.

In my room in
Susannah's apartment
there was a drawer
in an antique desk
where I kept the keys
to Sara's house.

I wasn't ready
to return them.
Sara was gone but
I wanted to keep
the possibility of
visiting her house
walking Lucky
making coffee
sitting on the sofa.

But at the same time
I knew in my heart
that going to Linden
was somehow wrong.

At best it was selfish
to give Lucky hope
that I would continue
to be part of his life.

At worst it was unsound
to hold on to Sara
through holding on to
her dog and her home

and all of her things
which included
my mother's things.

That was when
I remembered Elaine
that sad summer
after my mother's death
when Elaine showed up
at my mother's house
at least once a week
always with Henry
the smelliest shih tzu
in the entire world.

Only after Sara's death
did I realize Elaine
was simply following
the sorrow bird's song
to my mother's house
so she could touch
the remaining echoes
of her beautiful friend.

If only I had understood!
I would have given Elaine
a big hug and said
'I miss my mother too.
She's everywhere
in this house
but at the same time
she's nowhere.
It's not enough
but it's all we have.
Please come here
and be with her
as often as you like.'


**B**efore leaving for London
I met Sara's daughters
at the Westfield Diner.

I hadn't seen Vickie
since Sara's mass
and the last time

I saw Little Sarah
was outside Trader Joe's.
They had been busy
with their mother's estate
and they were wrestling
with their own sorrow birds.

Now I was the one
about to disappear
and we wanted to meet
before that happened.

It was still forbidden
to gather inside
so we sat underneath
the large event tent
in the parking lot
and ordered our lunch.

Life seemed impossible
after Sara's death.
But look!
We were sitting
at a restaurant.
We could eat
and we could talk.

Here we were
and we were alive.


**O**ur discussion was deep.
I told them my theory
that all of us had
experienced trauma
especially them.

I said my anger
and difficulty being
with other people
made me think
I was suffering from
some kind of PTSD.

Maybe mourning
was not just about
processing loss.

Maybe you also needed
to process trauma
particularly if you lost
someone in the way
we lost our Sara.

They agreed and
shared with me
their own stories
of life after Sara.

We also acknowledged
that Sara's death
had surely come
as a release for her
because her pain
was finally over.
As was the suffering
we experienced
while witnessing
Sara's agony.

But now our pain
had been replaced
with a new pain.
A black hole
in our centers
screaming with
the sound of no Sara.

Now we longed
for any Sara at all.
Mostly we yearned
for healthy Sara.
But we would also
have settled for
last summer's
half-healthy Sara.
Or even very ill Sara
who was confused
and couldn't walk
or feed herself.
We even wanted
that Sara back.

It was only now
when Sara was gone
we finally understood
that Sara had always
been Sara.

As lunch wound down
we talked about plans
for the future.

Vickie intended to
gradually
go back to her job.
Little Sarah planned to
gradually
study and work online
until it was possible
to return to Cornell.
And I of course
was on my way
to London.

When the waitress
gave us the check
I suddenly felt
a warm sense
of completion.

I had promised
to stay with Sara
until the end
and I had kept
my promise.

It's true I got wobbly
in the beginning
of the pandemic
when I tried to get
permission to stay
in Sweden.

It was probably time
to forgive myself
for that aberration.
And time once again

to acknowledge
what a gift it was
that the Universe
brought me back
to the only place
I needed to be.

Thanks Universe.

When it was time
to say goodbye
I reached into my purse
and pulled out the keys.

The girls insisted
it wasn't necessary
but I explained
why it actually was.

They nodded and
pocketed the keys.
Now my hands
were empty for real.

I watched the girls
as they walked
slowly to their car.
Strong and sad
mature and beautiful
courageous and kind.

They had gone through
something so painful
at such a young age.
And they had survived.

Sara's girls!
They were my heroines.

Thank you Vickie.
Thank you Little Sarah.

As for me
I had also survived.

Now life was once again
setting me on my feet
suitcase in hand
and sending me out
into the big unknown.

# Autumn/Winter 2020–21

Just like that
I was in London.

The trip overseas
wasn't complicated.
In September 2020
you didn't need
to take a covid test
or show paperwork
to fly from the US
to Great Britain.

The airport was
almost empty
and the plane itself
had few passengers.
Once again
I stretched out
over an entire row.

During that period
of the pandemic
travelers arriving
in Great Britain
had to quarantine
for 14 days
so I booked a hotel
with a quarantine packet
for overseas travelers.

Mostly I stayed
in my room
on the fourth floor
but I got to eat
in the hotel's café
on the ground floor.
A table in the corner
was set aside for
those in quarantine.

Sometimes I walked
round and round
the empty corridors

of the fourth floor
without ever seeing
a single living soul.

The staff told me
I could visit
the tiny park
across the street
as long as I had
a face mask on
and didn't interact
with anyone else.

Like a rat in a cage
I circled around
that patch of green
three times a day
looking longingly
at the world outside
the black iron gates
surrounding the park.

I could see the top
of The Gherkin
the spiral building
that resembles a pickle.
I promised myself
I would go there
just as soon as
quarantine was over.

Across the street I saw
a fish-and-chips shop
called Jack the Chipper.
I promised myself
I would eat there
just as soon as
I was free.

One Sunday morning
the park was empty.
Since there was no one
I could possibly infect
I sat on a large rock

and enjoyed some
much needed fresh air.

Which is when
a man all in black
stormed into the park
and started running
straight toward me
screaming furiously
'You don't belong here!'

I leapt up and ran
back to my hotel
with the crazy man
tight at my heels
still yelling at me
telling me something
I already knew.


Quarantine was
trying of course
but as the days passed
with books and naps
movies and yoga
the hotel became
a peaceful sanctuary
which allowed me
to recover from
my grueling summer.

Of course I was not
alone in my room.
The sorrow bird had
flown over with me.

Just like me
the sorrow bird
was shocked
to find itself
in a new nest
in a foreign city.

Just like me
the sorrow bird
was surprised

our new shelter
felt so healing.

There was however
one place in the hotel
that was not safe
namely my own mind.

The problem
was a raging case
of hypochondria
which kicked off
my last week in NJ.

At a normal checkup
to update my glasses
the optometrist asked
if I wanted a scan from
a fancy new machine.

'Sure' I said naively.

Afterward we inspected
creepy images of
the inside of my eyes
a bright orange mass
with a curling tangle
of black blood vessels.

My optician showed me
all the good things.
No macular degeneration
like my mother.
No cataracts
no glaucoma.

'And then'
she said
'we have this.'

She pointed at
a black spot.

My heart froze.
I stammered
'That doesn't look good.'

She replied
'I want a specialist
to run some tests.'

Immediately
I understood
what was going on.

Now it was my turn.
Now it was me
who had cancer.

Forget London.
Forget the future.
Just a long death
in a hospital bed
in a NJ suburb
just like Sara.

Now it was my turn.

It was no consolation
when the optometrist
said the black spot
could be nothing.

I knew from experience
that a test could confirm
your very worst fears.

It had happened to Sara
and now it was my turn.

**A** week passed
before I could meet
with the specialist.

During that time
I found it impossible
not to think about
the little black spot.

That week my heart
pounded feverishly
and my brain burned
with white-hot hysteria.

There were times
at most 15 minutes
when I was able to stop
thinking about the spot.

Listening to Natthiko
helped as always
although I knew
he had also gotten
his own horrible news
namely an ALS diagnosis.

But no matter
how much I tried
to distract myself
the sorrow bird
kept resurfacing
screeching at me
about my eye
and saying I had
a fatal illness
just like Sara.

I held my breath
for seven long days.

As I stepped into
the specialist's office
panic rippled
along my spine.

I went through
examination
after examination
frozen with fright.

And guess what?
Everything was OK.
More or less.

The doctor told me
I had a benign mole
on the back wall
of my left eye.

He also said
90 percent of
these kind of moles
never become cancer.

Good news.
But the adrenaline
had already rushed
so long and so fast
that I was unable
to wind down.

This happened
a few days before
I left for London
and unfortunately
that adrenaline
traveled with me.


Hypochondria had
seared a pathway
through my neurons
and once in quarantine
it started searching
for a new illness.

In my hotel room
I read a book
by Siri Hustvedt
where a character
gets diagnosed with
ovarian cancer.

As I read about
the character's symptoms
it became clear to me
I also suffered from
ovarian cancer.

I lay in bed and
shook with fear.
Now it was my turn.

My thoughts rushed
in a frantic torrent.
I planned to stay

in London
until March 1.
Should I return
to the US now
and visit a doctor?
But if I did
would I be
stuck in NJ
for treatment?

No no no!
Going back
felt impossible.
I needed a break
from sad empty NJ.

I decided to wait
until January
when I would get
my ovaries checked
by a London doctor.

I wanted
a final period
of normal life
before I became
a permanent patient
just like Sara.

Now it was my turn.
It had been Sara's turn
and now it was mine.

Simple and logical
in my mind anyway.

I only hoped that
I could face my illness
with the same courage
and dignity as Sara.

Sara my Sara.

The 14 days passed.
Finally I was released
from my quarantine cage.

The longed-for freedom
didn't feel as good
as I had imagined.

Suddenly
I found myself
in a strange city
moving too fast
in the wrong direction.

That first morning
during my short walk
to the Gherkin
I was almost run over
at least a dozen times.

As planned I ate
at Jack the Chipper
and nearly fainted
when I was served
a piece of fish
as big as my face.
Being moderate
which was so valued
in Swedish culture
was clearly not a priority
in this country.

Too unsettled to walk
or take the subway
I took a pricey taxi
and moved into
my Airbnb room
in Marylebone.

The sorrow bird
followed me there.

In its beak
it held a suitcase
full of mourning
and on its back
it bore a knapsack
crammed full
with hypochondria.

The first three weeks
out of quarantine
when I wasn't busy
dodging British traffic
I bristled inwardly
at all the differences
between London
and Stockholm.

The coffee in London
was tasteless.
The people in London
were loud.
The streets in London
were dirty.
And did I mention
everything was moving
in the wrong direction?

Covid was increasing
in London just then
and I was full of fear.
Too afraid even
to travel on the tube
or a charming red bus.

Instead I took
long lonely walks
in Marylebone.
I needed to move
so I could hold at bay
the obsessive thoughts
about ovarian cancer
shouting in my head.

I missed Sara.
I missed Sweden.
I missed all my friends
who were strewn
all over the world
with not a single one
in London.

I felt more lost
and frightened
than ever before.

The sorrow bird
sang incessantly.
A shrill song
just as loud
if not louder
than in NJ.

The only difference
was now it sang
in a British accent.

What I didn't know
was that a miracle
was approaching.

Several actually.

As it says in the famous
Native American proverb:
Give thanks for
unknown blessings
already on their way.

London was where
the Universe stopped
taking away my friends
and instead started
giving me new ones.

Filled up my life
instead of emptying it.

The new era began
when my loneliness
and hypochondria
finally impelled me
to attend online
12-step meetings
as well as other
cyber activities.

During one such gathering
I told the digital strangers
I was in London
alone in quarantine.

A few minutes later
a private message
popped up on my screen:
Florence my name is Berlin.
I'm from Australia
and I know how it feels
to be new in London.
When quarantine is over
let's get a coffee.

A few weeks later
during an online
Swedish get-together
I told the digital strangers
I was in London
and missed Stockholm.

A few minutes later
a private message
popped up on my screen:
Florence my name is Kristina.
I'm in London and
I also miss Stockholm.
Do you want to get a coffee?

I met Berlin at
Fischer's in Marylebone
one of Karl Ove Knausgård's
favorite restaurants.

When I asked Berlin
'How will I recognize you?'
she answered
'I'm tall with pink hair.'

Berlin and I
discovered we had
a lot in common
including writing.
We clicked.

I met Kristina
in Fitzrovia
at a Swedish café
called Fabrique.

We realized at once
we had actually met
before in Stockholm
the previous spring.
We clicked.

Life took my Sara from me
but then it gave me
an Australian named Berlin
and a Swede named Kristina
who I already knew.

As if life was applying
a soothing balm
to my sunburned heart.


The Swedish Church
was another gift.

The first time
I entered the church
with its high ceiling
thick stone walls and
elegant stained glass
I saw these words
on the altar wall:
God is love.

The message hit my heart
direct and intense.
It was simple
without doctrine
available for all
including me
a disoriented American
with a passionate love
for all things Swedish.
It clicked.

After the service
I went to fellowship

in the common room.
As I eagerly drank
strong Swedish coffee
everyone around me
was extremely willing
to chat and connect.

That was when
I experienced firsthand
the deep groove of isolation
etched into the English soul
after their first and
most brutal lockdown.

I continued going to services
and during the weekdays
I visited the church café
where the young volunteers
Carolina and Isak
served strong coffee and
fresh cinnamon buns
with plenty of time
for a chat in Swedish.

After a few weeks
attending the church
I felt like an imposter
since I was not Christian.
I booked a meeting
with Deacon Helen
to discuss my conflict.

On a weekday afternoon
we met in a little room
just off the chapel.
Helen listened carefully
as I told her about
my journey with
and away from
Christianity.

I took a deep breath
and asked her
'Can I come here
even if I don't

accept everything
or actually
almost nothing?'

Helen looked me
straight in the eye.
'If you like coming here
then just come.'

She also said
if I would like
we could meet
once a week
and have a talk.

I said yes at once.

The next week
we met again
in the silent church.
I told Helen
about my Sara
and everything that
I had witnessed
Sara endure.
I said how much
Sara's suffering
still plagued me
and how rootless
I had been feeling
since her death.

The next time we met
Helen carried out
a private ceremony
simple and modest
for both Sara and me.
A calming rain
on the raw flames
of my grief.

Life had taken away
my childhood home
but during those weeks
it gave me back
a spiritual home.

Another gift was
the online school
Swedish Made Easy
led by Anneli and Daniel
two Swedes residing
in Great Britain.

Since the school
took place online
it didn't matter
where anyone lived
but I liked the fact
that my teachers
were also in the UK.
It was fun discussing
British culture and
corona politics
in Swedish.

The school offered
a language café
Wednesday evenings.
I started attending
and just like that
I had a digital gang
to hang out with.
It clicked.

That's where I met
the Englishman David
who played violin and
the Swedish nyckelharpa.
He lived in London
so we decided
to meet in real life
and speak Swedish.

We met at Bageriet
a cozy Swedish bakery
hidden in an alleyway
near Covent Garden.
Due to the pandemic
we were only allowed
to sit outside in the cold
so we huddled around

a little wooden table
drinking strong coffee
and eating princess cake.

David helped me feel
at home in Great Britain.
At the same time
he helped keep alive
my connection to
Sweden and Swedish.

One day I happened
to look at Bageriet's
Instagram account.
A picture showed
two people sitting
outside the bakery
on a winter evening
deep in conversation.
A cozy little scene
with golden light
from Bageriet's window
shining on the two friends.

Suddenly I realized
I was looking at
a photograph of
David and me.

Life had taken
Sweden from me
including my friends
and our conversations
over cake and coffee.
But now it gave me
a lovely group
of online friends.

Life also gave me
a physical friend
with whom I could
drink strong coffee
in a London alleyway
fragrant with the aroma
of fresh-baked cinnamon buns.

In November
I discovered
the crown jewel
of life in London.

There were precious few
in-person 12-step meetings
in London just then
but I heard about
a meeting in Soho
at St. Anne's Church
on Dean Street
every morning at 7.30.

I rarely attend
morning meetings
since that's when
I like to write.
But I needed
12-step desperately
so I decided to go.

On November 5
the first day of Britain's
second national lockdown
I went to the meeting
for the first time.

I was the only person
sitting in the tube
and I was all alone
walking through Soho
along Shaftesbury Avenue
past shuttered theaters.

I turned left
onto Dean Street.
Halfway down the block
I saw a little group
huddled together.

The thought arose:
There they are.

As if I already
knew them.

As if this was
a reunion.
It clicked.

The meeting room
had large windows
a crystal chandelier
wood-paneled walls
and a painting of
a stern Englishman
in a high white collar.
Everyone called it
the Harry Potter room.

I went to the meeting
every morning
and almost every time
I spoke of Sara.

I also shared about
the hypochondria
racing in my brain.

Everyone listened
intently to me
and I listened
intently to them.

Physical meetings
had a strict limit
of 17 people.
Each of us had
a sorrow bird
and fortunately
the Harry Potter room
had space for them too.

Which is when
I discovered that
the sorrow bird
is a flock animal.
Who knew?

Life had taken away
my 12-step meetings
in NJ and Stockholm

but then it gave me
a new home group
with new people
who I felt as if
I already knew.

**B**ritain's second lockdown
was actually the first one
I had ever experienced.

The streets were empty.
Most stores were closed.
You could buy drinks
and food to take away
but you were not allowed
to drink and eat inside.
All public toilets
were firmly closed.

Big signs were propped
at the entrance of
every tube station.
Angry red letters
shouted that only those
with a valid reason
were allowed to travel.

Happily I had one!
Support-group members
were thankfully included
on the list of exceptions.

The lockdown
was undoubtedly
a hell for many and
one mustn't forget that.
But for me just then
the locked-down world
was a peaceful adventure.

London was mine!
I had the city to myself
those tranquil mornings
riding an empty tube car

or walking 40 minutes
from Marylebone to Soho.

No matter how I traveled
I always passed through
Piccadilly Circus
London's beating heart
which at that time
barely had a pulse.

Before the meeting
I chatted with the others
outside St. Anne's.
After the meeting
we all walked over
to St. Giles' churchyard
and drank coffee from
the kiosk Rosie & Joe
run by a kind man
named Andrew.

On those cold
November mornings
our group huddled
together outside
talking and laughing
for at least an hour
sometimes longer.

Everyone was on furlough
so no one had a job
they had to go to.

Everything was closed
so no one had appointments
they needed to keep.

We had nothing
except each other
and that was enough.

In the afternoons
during lockdown
I often met
Berlin or Kristina
or a 12-step friend

to do the only thing
you could do then
namely go on a walk
in an empty park
carrying a cup
of take-away tea.

That was also when
Swedish Made Easy
had a four-week course
with a Zoom seminar
on Wednesday evenings.
I looked forward to
those weekly seminars
like a child yearns
for Christmas.

Bageriet was allowed
to stay open for take-out
so I still met David
in the hidden alleyway
and spoke Swedish
while drinking coffee
and eating princess cake.

Even though London
was in lockdown
I was not isolated
and I was not alone.

That was a gift.

One day in November
I was walking through
the locked-down city
and I suddenly felt
an odd sensation
in my chest.

I couldn't fathom
what was happening.
I stood still and
tried to figure out
what I was feeling.

Then I realized
I was happy.

Because the feeling
had been absent
so many months
I hadn't recognized it
when it finally returned.

I was happy
standing in the heart
of an empty city
in a foreign country
that had embraced me.

The happiness
blooming in my chest
was a fine surprise
that sent tears of joy
to my open eyes.

Naturally
I wasn't happy
the entire time
during lockdown.

Sometimes the sorrow bird
shrieked songs of hypochondria
disturbing the quiet party
of life in lockdown London.

At times the only thing
I could think about was
the upcoming doctor visit
to check my ovaries.

But I had my daily
12-step meetings
where I could share
thoughts and fears
about my hypochondria.
It helped to say aloud
how terrified I was
how racing and fearful
my thoughts had become.

People at the meetings
couldn't take away
my hypochondria
but they could
walk beside me
as I went through it
and that's what they did.

The Swedish Church
was unfortunately closed
but on Sunday afternoons
we had online gatherings
which was also something
I eagerly looked forward to.

Otherwise I stayed home
in quiet Marylebone.
The little Edwardian house
where I rented a room
had no other guests
due to the lockdown
so I had the place
all to myself.

I filled my days
with writing
Natthiko talks
Swedish studies
British detective series
and long deep naps
in the silent house.

Everything helped
my sunburned heart
regain its strength
and come back to life.

London November 2020.
A chilly autumn
calm and still
with the empty silence
of a barren city
holding its breath.

Of course
I never forgot Sara.

Of course not.
I thought of her
every single day.

When my birthday
came around
I knew that hers
would be arriving
three days later.

On Sara's birthday
her friend Paula
shared pictures of her
on Facebook and wrote
'Now all we have left
are photos and memories.'

When I read that
I cried.

I realized that
if those things
were indeed
all we had left
of my Sara
then we needed
to hold on to them
as tight as we could.

Sara's birthday
remained
Sara's birthday
even if she no longer
was there to celebrate.

Happy birthday
my beautiful friend!

Britain came out of
its second lockdown
on December 2.

Soon after
covid cases
rose sharply.
New restrictions
were imposed
and the shops
had to close
just a few weeks
before Christmas.

The disappointment
was palpable.
A fog of sorrow
fell over the city.
It felt as if Christmas
had been canceled.

There were however
points of light.
My meetings
remained untouched.
Bageriet was thankfully
still in business.
The Swedish Church
managed to stay open
in a limited fashion
with holiday concerts
and a Christmas market.

I invited Berlin and Kristina
and a new friend
named Suzanne
to the Christmas market.
We visited the booths
and stocked up on
shrimp sandwiches
princess cake slices
and saffron buns.

Back at my house
we set out our feast
in the living room.
We ate Swedish food
drank tea and coffee

talked and laughed
the whole afternoon.

A year later
I went to therapy
and the therapist asked
if I could remember
a time when I was
particularly happy.

Immediately I recalled
that joyful afternoon
in Marylebone
December 2020.

Even though London
was slipping back into
yet another lockdown
I was not isolated
and I was not alone.

That was a gift.

Christmas Day
was lovely.

In the morning
I walked to my meeting
happy and grateful.

The streets were empty
as I strolled from
Marylebone to Soho.
The rare times
I saw someone
I called out cheerfully
'Merry Christmas!'

That worked well
with big smiles and
Christmas greetings back
until a guy on a bicycle
turned around and
started following me.

Oy!
London was a wild beast
even on Christmas Day.

I shook him off
and stopped greeting
the people I passed by.
Or rather I ceased
greeting them aloud
and instead hailed them
silently in my heart.

Silent
exactly like
the rest of the city.

Merry Christmas London!

January 1 2021
was the day when
Brexit became official.

A rainy day which
I spent with Tom
and Ed the Blonder
in Highgate Cemetery.
We had a lovely time
but a pall hung
over the country
as if someone
or something
had died.

January 6 2021
Great Britain started
its third lockdown.

The atmosphere
felt more serious
than it had during
November's lockdown.
You could only socialize
with one other household
and police lurked
in the London streets

looking for anyone
breaking the rules.

A fear had crept in
regardless of
where you were
regardless of
what you did.

Thank goodness
my 12-step meeting
continued as usual.
Many cafés and
restaurants were
open for take-out.
But otherwise
everything was closed.

One time Tom and I
and curly-haired Christina
went to Russell Square.
We had a conversation
with our backs
turned to one another
concealing our friendship
from a nearby policeman.

One time after
a 12-step meeting
a little group of us
broke the rules
and stood in front
of Caffè Nero
on Frith Street.

When someone
yelled 'Police!'
we ran frantically
in opposite directions
disappearing into
the streets of London
like a gang of pickpockets
from Oliver Twist.

London was not
quite as much fun

now that socializing
was a crime.

The third lockdown
wasn't the only thing
creating a serious tone
during those weeks.

Finally it was time
to visit the doctor
and check my ovaries.

As I sat on the cold
examination table
in a blue paper gown
my inhalations
were long and shaky.

When the doctor
did the ultrasound
he burst out
'Your ovaries
are so tiny!'

No cancer.
No nothing.
All my symptoms
turned out to be
a complete fantasy.

I was relieved
but unfortunately
my deliverance was fragile.
Despite the good news
my veins still pulsed
with the frenzied dread
of hypochondria.

My next health check
was at The Mole Clinic.

A few years earlier
I had a benign spot
burned off my forehead.
My dermatologist

told me I needed
an annual scan
so I booked one
in central London.

Everything went well
till the nurse looked
at my right foot.
Between my toes
she found a red patch
which I knew about
since it had been there
as long as I could remember.

The nurse took
several pictures
to be examined
by a specialist.

Two days later
I got an email
which said that
the red spot was
extremely uneven
and I was to come
back for a biopsy.
They even used
the word urgent.

I read the email
as I was leaving
my 12-step meeting.
I got tunnel vision
and my friends' voices
seemed to come from
very far away.

Now it was my turn.
Now I had cancer
just like Sara.

I booked a biopsy.
Immediately afterward
I called Berlin.

Because of corona
no one was allowed
to accompany you
into the clinic
so Berlin promised
to wait for me
right outside.

In the days
before the procedure
my brain burned with
catastrophic thoughts.

At my daily meeting
I shared about
my upcoming biopsy.
A temporary relief
in the middle of
my boiling anxiety.

Finally it was time
for the appointment.
My sight was blurry
from racing panic
and every second
felt like a year.

The doctor who
took the biopsy
said the mark
appeared to be
a harmless clump
of burst blood vessels.

A week later
I got the results.
Sure enough
the red patch
was benign.

The most important thing
I took from that experience
was not the good news.
It was rather how I felt
when I came outside
after the biopsy and

saw Berlin standing
in her fake fur coat
on Argyll Street
on a cold Saturday
in lockdown London.

Berlin couldn't take away
what was happening to me.
All she could do
was walk beside me
while I went through it.
Which she did.

Thanks Berlin.


**A**merican tourists
are allowed to stay
in Great Britain
six months at a time.

I planned to leave
on March 1
exactly six months
after I had arrived.

My next country
would be Ireland
where I would
wait for Sweden
to open up again.

A good plan
that collapsed
due to Delta
a covid strain
spreading quickly
in Great Britian.

Suddenly I was
in the epicenter
of a dangerous
new mutation.

Almost overnight
all countries refused
to welcome tourists

coming from
Great Britain.
Namely me.

My six months were
coming to a close
and I had to leave.
I could have applied
for an extension
but after my rejection
from Swedish immigration
I was reluctant to try.

Once again
only one country
was willing to take me
namely the land
of my passport.

Once again
the nearest exit
was behind me.


**I** said goodbye
to my new friends
the Swedish Church
my 12-step meeting
beautiful Bageriet
lovely London.

I promised to return
as soon as I could.

I traveled on
an almost empty tube
which took me to
an almost empty airport.
When I boarded
an almost empty plane
I stretched out over
an entire row.

That plane
flew me back
to the place where
I didn't want to go.

# Winter/Spring 2021

In Westfield
once again.

As the taxi driver
drove into town
I leaned forward
ready to tell him
to turn right toward
my mother's house.

The sorrow bird
swooped closer
whispering that
my mother was
no longer there
and the house
now belonged
to another family.

I sat back
in my seat
and stayed mute.


In the beginning
I was in quarantine
for two weeks.

When I was free
I once again entered
a restricted world.
Westfield had
no 12-step meetings
no yoga classes
and still so much
free-floating fear
due to the pandemic.

Without my mother
and without Sara
the air felt thin.
As if every breath
fell short of full.

A lonesome feeling
to once again
step into nothing.

But despite the
stifling emptiness
Westfield was still
my only real home
in my homeland.

Anywhere else
would have been
even emptier.

Despite everything
there was an extremely
positive development.

Sweden had new rules.
Regardless of citizenship
anyone could enter Sweden
if they traveled there
from an EU country.

Only problem was
no EU countries
were currently open
to American tourists.

I needed to continue
waiting in Westfield
until some country
just one country
unlocked its border.

Several times a day
I checked the news
and my Facebook groups.

Rumor had it
Croatia would soon
open up for tourism.
When that happened
I could fly there and
travel on to Sweden.

On the mirror
in my room
I taped up a quote
from The I Ching:

In a great storm
the wise bird
returns to her nest
and waits patiently.


One advantage to
being back in NJ
was taking care of
practical things
I couldn't do overseas.

I renewed my passport
for another ten years.
I visited multiple doctors
despite every examination
igniting my hypochondria.

I worked on my short stories
every single day.
I had online Swedish lessons
a few times a week.

That season of waiting
was not without
its small pleasures.
You could now sit inside
cafés and restaurants
which meant I could
meet my friends
for coffee or dinner.

Every encounter
with every friend
was a ray of light
in an otherwise
monotone existence.

An unexpected gift
was a newly formed
12-step meeting

in a nature reserve
about 30 minutes
from where I lived.
I had no car
but now and then
I got a lift.

It was healing
to spend time with
my 12-step friends
who I had seen
nearly every day
during the years
I lived in NJ
with my mother.

Each person
was a shining star
beautiful and fine.

We met one another
in the nature reserve
at a social distance
but we walked
beside one another
as close as we could.

One person
I saw regularly
was Little Sarah.

Such a joy meeting her at
Boxwood Coffee Roasters
in downtown Westfield
and talking eagerly about
books and psychology
politics and philosophy
her plans and my plans
and of course
her mother
our Sara.

Two moments
with Little Sarah

stand out as
especially radiant.

One was when
Little Sarah sat
across from me
and I was struck
by how much she
resembled her mother.

Time fell away
and suddenly
I saw Sara's face
looking back at me.

I blinked away
my joyful tears.
Just for a moment
I had seen Sara's face
and that was a sight
I had truly missed.

Another moment
was when Little Sarah
said that recently
she had experienced
a moment of clarity
when she was filled
with a feeling
deep down
clear and strong
that everything
was OK.

What had happened
had happened
and it was OK.

I understood
what she meant.
A sense that you
could live with
what had happened
because that's
what had happened.

350

Little Sarah
had so much faith
in life just then
so much strength
and lucid wisdom.
After everything
she and her family
had lived through
it was a pure miracle
to hear her say that.

That was her truth
and I hoped one day
it might be mine.


**I** saw Lucky
one last time.

A short visit to
use the bathroom
in Sara's house
after a day trip
to Woodstock
with Little Sarah.

It was strange
but not unpleasant
to once again
find myself
in Sara's house.

The sorrow bird
was still there
filling the air with
a melancholy hum.

I hadn't seen Lucky
for nine months
but he fell at once
into our old pattern.

First he went berserk
and I bent down
so I could pet him.
He glared at me
while I talked

with Little Sarah.
A few minutes later
he got impatient and
started clawing me
letting me know
it was time for our walk!

But there was no time
for our walk.
It was evening and
I was only there
for a short visit.

As I moved toward
the front door
without the leash
and without him
Lucky stood still
and watched me with
a perplexed expression.

Why won't you walk me?
Why aren't you staying?
Please don't go.

My little friend.
The very best dog
in the entire world
who gave so much love
to my mother and Sara
and both their families.

A rescue dog
who rescued us.


Like a hawk
I checked the news
and my travel groups
several times a day
desperate for a sign
that Croatia had lifted
its travel restrictions.

Mid-April 2021
while eating lunch
with Little Sarah

at Bare Burger
in Westfield
my phone pinged.

A Croatian travel agency
had sent an email
declaring the country
was now open for
American tourists!

Unfortunately
there was a catch.
To travel to Croatia
I needed to show
a negative covid test
taken 48 hours
before my arrival.
But during that stage
of the pandemic
covid tests took
at least 72 hours
before you got the results.

Luckily Little Sarah
knew about a drugstore
in a large supermarket
where I could get
a 15-minute test.

The day before my flight
I went to the drugstore.
A technician stuck
a long cotton swab
inside my throat and
twirled another swab
inside my nostrils.

For 15 long minutes
I paced the store
praying that my future
could finally begin.

The test was negative
thank goodness.

April 2021
I flew away
from the US
and I haven't
been back
since then.

Goodbye.

# Spring 2021 to Spring 2022

When Chögyam Trungpa Rinpoche
was forced to leave Tibet after
the Chinese invasion in 1959
he wrote a poem called Stray Dog.

The first lines read:
Chögyam is merely a stray dog.
He wanders around the world.

During the next year
I thought often of those lines
but I changed them to:
Florence is merely a stray dog.
She wanders around the world.

Obviously I was not
a refugee like he was.
I was a retired American
with a valid passport
and my departure
had been voluntary.

What I was experiencing
was an exile of the heart.
Because the place
my heart had lived
with my mother and Sara
had ceased to exist
and I couldn't return.

Westfield was still there
but when I thought
about Westfield
it felt like a desert
flat and barren with
a bleak whistling wind
of the sorrow bird's howl.


The next 16 months
looked like this:

April to May 2021
Croatia
(Zagreb and Split)

June to August 2021
Stockholm
(Finally! After 379 days
in travel-restriction exile)

September to November 2021
London
(Again! Hurrah!)

December 2021
Dublin

January to March 2022
Stockholm

April to June 2022
London

July 2022
(Right now when
I'm writing these words)
Dublin and Spain


This lifestyle was
not as unstable
as it might sound.

For many years
Sweden had been
my second home.
As soon as I arrived
I slipped into
my Swedish life.
Same room at
the same hotel
same friends in
the same cafés
and 12-step meetings.

It was also like that
in Great Britain
which had become
my *second* second home.

I had no residency
in those countries
but I had a full life
in each of them.

I longed to live
in one country.
Unfortunately
I didn't want
to live in the country
I was allowed to live in.
And I wasn't allowed
to live in the countries
I wanted to live in.

A first-world problem
in every respect.

Regardless of
where I found myself
I worked diligently
on my short stories
and my Swedish.

I didn't miss
a single day.

Sara accompanied me
in those activities as well.
The short story collection
was dedicated to her and
there was even a story
about brain cancer.

My writing and
Swedish studies
wove through
every country
like a red thread
holding me together
and creating a daily life
I could count on.

A strategy for
creating stability
in instability.

This was however
a brittle lifestyle.
So many things
could go wrong.

A pandemic
could break out
and borders could
close overnight.

Someone at
passport control
could mistrust me
and block my entry.

Staying just one day
over my 90 tourist days
could lead to being
expelled from Europe
for a whole year.

Another problem
with this way of life
was my difficulty
explaining it to others.

In Stockholm
two Tinder dates
crashed and burned
because the men
questioned me
in a judgmental way
about my lifestyle.

Both dates took place
at Vete-Katten café.
Each time I made
an excuse midway
and went to hide
in the toilet.

The second time
I texted my friend Fanny.
Help! I wrote.
I am on the world's
worst Tinder date!

Fanny wrote back:
Leave!
So I did.

Those men thought
my way of life
was strange
rather frivolous
definitely unreliable.

But listen guys!
That isn't true at all!
I am merely a stray dog.
I wander around the world.

Woof woof!

February 2022
I published my short stories
Annikas Förråd (in Swedish)
Annika's Storage Space (in English).

A few months later
in Stockholm
I finally finished
marketing the books.

Suddenly I had
nothing to edit
nothing to translate
nothing to proofread.

No more books to mail
no more emails to send
no more articles to write
no more podcasts to tape.

One evening
I was lying in bed
in my hotel room
when to my surprise
I saw the sorrow bird
perched by my feet.

It stared at me with
enormous wise eyes
and sang this song:

Are you finally ready
to stop running
so you can listen
to my lament?

That's when I realized
the sorrow bird had
never stopped warbling.
It was rather that
I had tried to fly away
from the sorrow bird
both physically
and psychically.

But it didn't work
because you can't avoid
the sorrow bird's hymns.
Not with
sex
food
work
drugs
travel
alcohol
exercise
TV series
socializing.

You can of course try!
But the sorrow bird
is stronger than
all those escapes
with a patience
endless as time.
It sings its ballads
despite what you do
or don't do.

The entire time
I was frantically
working on my books
and studying Swedish
the sorrow bird
had waited for me.

Nothing had thawed.
Nothing had vanished.
My sadness was
stronger than ever.

It took time before
I finally was ready
to stop everything and
listen to the sorrow bird.

After Stockholm
I traveled to London
where I distracted myself
a few months longer.

June 2022
I arrived in Dublin
and moved into a hotel
in a calm neighborhood.

A corner room
big and fresh
sparsely furnished
with large windows
overlooking a canal
with lots of light
when it wasn't raining.
Plenty of space
for both me and
the sorrow bird.

Every morning
I sat upright
in the roomy bed
with large soft pillows
and bright white sheets
and wrote this book.

During those mornings
I didn't write for long
maybe an hour max.
And I didn't write much
just two or three pages.
That was all I could bear.

I gave my life over
to the sorrow bird.

I put its needs
first and foremost.

I left space
for its song.

I'm not saying
it was easy.
While I wrote
I cried often
and hard.

But what a relief
to finally stop running!
Who knew it could be
so incredibly healing
just to stay still
and listen?


When I wasn't writing
I did very little.

I went to 12-step meetings
and took long walks
but mostly I lay in bed
read detective novels
listened to podcasts
watched films and series
mostly Irish ones
including Sally Rooney's
Normal People and
Conversations with Friends.

Dublin itself was
a pleasant surprise.
Every day I walked
to my 12-step meeting
through St. Stephen's Green
with its colorful flowers
and aggressive seagulls
who once plucked a croissant
right out of my hand.

Regardless of where
I was in Dublin
it felt like I was living
inside a Sally Rooney book.

And what joy
when one day
I actually saw her!
She was walking along
St. Stephen's Green
a normal person
having a conversation
with a friend.

I was totally starstruck.
Out of respect
I didn't follow her
although I certainly
was sorely tempted.

In short
I enjoyed Dublin
and I liked the Irish
who underneath
their social warmth
and lively chattiness
carry a painful history.
Every person
in that country
knows the sorrow bird
all too well.


**M**y 12-step meeting
was on Clarendon Street
beside St. Teresa's Church.
A church for both
St. Teresa of Avila and
St. Therese of Lisieux.

Little Therese again!
Every day before
my midday meeting
I went to her altar
and lit a votive candle.
I kneeled down and

thanked Little Therese
for helping me with
that day's writing
and asked for help
for the next day too.

It felt as if Little Therese
carried me while
I wrote this book.
I doubt I could have
done it without her.

It's only fair to wonder
if I actually got help
from Little Therese.
My answer is:
It doesn't matter if it's true.
The most important thing
is that it worked.

Which it did.
Otherwise
how could you possibly
be reading this now?


During those days
writing in Dublin
Lucky died.

He was old
and he was sick.
It was his time.

A sad day
when Vickie called
to give me the news.

Now the pact between
my mother and Sara
had been honored.

Now Frank's promise
that Lucky would be loved
until the day he died
was also fulfilled.

Vickie told me
the vet gave them
clay impressions of
Lucky's paw print.
Frank even got his
transferred into a tattoo.

That paw print
waits for me
in a drawer
in Vickie's house
in Linden NJ
far away from
where I am now.


Toward the end of
those days in Dublin
my hypochondria
finally subsided.

I searched throughout
my clean white room
but it was gone.

For the first time
I could think about
the hypochondria
with a bit of distance.

On the one hand
it was understandable.
Sara's illness taught me
worst fears can come true.
The pain in your stomach
might be ovarian cancer
and the spot on your retina
could be a degenerative disease.

A deadly illness is
always a possibility.
That's just life.
When you know that
it's not possible
to unknow it.

On the other hand
my hypochondria
was a way to mourn
or rather a result of
my refusal to mourn.

It was the sorrow bird
who created the fear
and intrusive thoughts.
It had hunted me
via the hypochondria
and refused to leave
until I dared sit still.

I also became aware
of yet another reason
for my hypochondria.

I was listening to
a Swedish podcast
with a Ukrainian woman.
She used the phrase
survivor's guilt
and the penny dropped.

That's what I had.
A habitual guilt
because it was Sara
who got sick
and not me.

Hypochondria
arose in part
from a strange need
to punish myself
because I was still here
and Sara was not.

Then I remembered
the 1980 film
Ordinary People
about a boy involved
in a boating accident
which he survived
and his brother did not.

At the end of the film
the boy understands
he survived because
he held on to the boat.
His brother couldn't
but the boy could
and so he did.

I did that too
or rather
my body did.
It held on
and it survived.

That's when I realized
that if I do get sick
it won't be because
Sara got sick.
My illness would
have nothing to do
with her illness.
They would be
two separate events.

My Sara got sick
and she died.
That's what happened.

As Little Sarah said
that day in Westfield:
It was OK.
What happened
had happened
and it was OK.

I could live with
what had happened
because that's
what had happened.

And my constant flight?
What was that about?

Was it merely bad luck
I didn't want to live
in the land I was

allowed to live in
and I wasn't allowed
to live in the lands
I wanted to live in?

Maybe.
Or maybe
it was because
when I imagined
going back to NJ
I got frightened
truly terrified
by the emptiness.

One night in Dublin
I dreamed I was back
at my mother's house.
I was in the garage
which was full to the brim
with furniture and objects
exactly as it had been
after my mother's death.

My mother was there
as were Sara and Lucky
and many others.

I stood in the middle
giving directions.
We were busy
but we were happy
because we were together.

All at once
the garage was empty
with bright white walls
and a shiny clean floor.

I stood in the center
of the empty garage
completely alone.

That hollow room
was the root of
my rootlessness.

Florence is merely a stray dog.
She wanders around the world.

Home is home.
But what do you do
if you have no home?

That sadly beautiful
period in Dublin
lasted 34 days.

It closed naturally
when I traveled to
Ourense Spain
at the end of July
for Vickie and
Jose's wedding.

To once again meet
Vickie and Little Sarah
and Sara's other friends
including Karla
was something I
eagerly anticipated.

The closest airport
to Ourense was
Santiago de Compostela
so I flew there.

I didn't know
Santiago de Compostela
is among the world's
most holy places.
The final destination
for seekers walking
an ancient pilgrimage route
called the Camino.

Once again I thought of
the Native American proverb:
Give thanks for
unknown blessings
already on their way.

Santiago de Compostela
is an ancient city with
an exquisite cathedral
white stone buildings
wide-open plazas and
winding back streets
full of tranquil shadows.

Pilgrims were everywhere.
As I sat in the shade
drinking cappuccinos
and eating churros
I was mesmerized
by the steady stream
of nomads walking past.

An astonishing mix
of ages and sizes
colors and genders
everyone equipped with
sturdy walking staffs
and thick kneepads
dusty hiking boots
and wide-brimmed hats
overstuffed backpacks
with a dangling metal cup.

Each pilgrim had just
survived a physical
and spiritual challenge
possibly unlike anything
they had previously endured.

Despite exhaustion
and heavy equipment
they exuded nobility.
Even those who limped
appeared to be strong
at least emotionally.

Sitting in the shade
it occurred to me
I had also completed
a kind of pilgrimage.

Like them I had just
survived a physical
and spiritual challenge
definitely unlike anything
I had previously endured.

I also limped
although my limp
was internal.

And yes I was
emotionally strong.

Yes.


The next day
before traveling
via train to Ourense
I woke up early
and took a walk.

The sun wasn't up
but night had receded
and the city was bathed
in a tender white light
from the coming dawn.

The gentle silence
was broken only
by delicate birdsong
and the timeless sound
of ringing church bells.

As I wandered through
the awakening city
I thought of Sara.
How I wished
I could meet her
later in Ourense.

Hello my dear!
Hello my beautiful friend!

How glad
we would have been
to meet up overseas!

How happy
she would have been
to be the mother of the bride!

But no matter how much
I wished to see Sara
it would never happen.

Sara was gone
and she had been gone
almost exactly two years.

There are certain facts in life
unyielding and hard as stone
which you can't ever change.

Sara's death
was one of them.

And yet as I
wandered around
the quietly dawning city
I realized something else.

Alongside everything
hard and brutal
there also exists
a dimension of life
fluid and invisible.

A private world
enclosed inside
our transparent hearts.

That's where
the ones we love
the ones we have lost
continue to live.

Of course Sara was
coming to the wedding!
Naturally she was invited
and I would carry her there.

In my heart's eye
I saw Sara wearing
a colorful dress

spiky high heels
a broad-brimmed hat
on her long bronze hair.
With that smile
wider than ever.
Mother of the bride.

The miraculous thing
was that her family
and many friends
would carry her too.

Sara wasn't gone!
She had multiplied.
And that's because
in the unseen world
there are no borders
and miracles flow daily.

Sara was still with us.
Luminously invisible
wonderfully iridescent.

There she goes!
Dancing through
waves of stardust.
Flying free
like a scent
a sunbeam
a symphony.

The sorrow bird
would also be coming
to Vickie's wedding.

Definitely not
an invited guest.
More like a gatecrasher.

No one wanted
the sorrow bird to sing.
But when had that ever
stopped a sorrow bird?

In Mio My Mio
Astrid Lindgren says

the sorrow bird
is big and black
with kind eyes.

In my experience
the sorrow bird
is a shape-shifter.
Frail as a hummingbird
common as a sparrow
callous as a hawk
stoic as an eagle.

Its songs also vary
shifting between
threatening screeches
melancholy choirs
pathetic moans
dramatic arias.

Sometimes
the sorrow bird
keeps perfectly still
hiding in dark corners
of menacing silence.

Sometimes
the sorrow bird
smashes into windows
that appear to be open
but are actually closed.

At Vickie's wedding
the sorrow bird
would once again
shift its shape.

Flying above the guests
feathers soft and white
with eyes composed of
two round diamonds.

A sparkling tiara
perched on its head
wingtips brushed
in liquid gold.

Gracing the air
with a gentle song
laced in sorrow.

The sun rose
above the city
white and clear
pure and strong.

I put on a hat and
smeared sunscreen
on my face and arms.

As I wandered
the curving streets
I felt light and free
as if something
was carrying me.

Was I being borne
by Christ energy?
This was after all
Santiago de Compostela
and it was no coincidence
the Camino pilgrimage
ended just here.

But wait!
Why should I limit
this precious energy
to Jesus Christ?
Holy energy
exists everywhere
Sin each culture
and every religion.

Whatever it was
I felt marvelous.
Never before
had I known
such lightness.
As if I could just
lift my arms and
rise into the sky!

And that was when
the light bulb went on.
I had drank three cups
of strong Spanish coffee.
Surely that was the source
of this special feeling.

A letdown to be sure.
But only for a moment.
It occurred to me
I didn't need to choose
between holy energy
or excess caffeine.
Perhaps the feeling
was a mixture of both?

It didn't matter
what was true.
The important thing
was that it worked.

And it did.
I was happy
and I felt free.


Glioblastoma
is a merciless way to die.

I think again about
what comedian
Per Andersson said:

Horrible things
happen in life.
That's just how it is.
But we were going
to try and push back.
We would give
life a fight.

I realized then
that holding on
to the invisible
is an excellent way
to push back.

Loving someone
we no longer see
is a superb way
of giving life a fight.

I have to do this
because if I don't
I find it impossible
to live this life
and I cannot cope
with all these losses.

But please!
Don't wait until
someone you love
suddenly receives
a devastating diagnosis.

Push back now!
Give life a fight
this very second!

And you know what?
Sara lived like that.
She was pushing back
and giving life a fight
all those moments
she lit up a room
with her big smile
and open heart.

O Sara!
Sara my Sara.

The listening is over.
Sara's book is done.

Here's another place
where Sara can live.
A memory palace
composed of words
where anyone at all
can visit my Sara.

But even though
the book ends here

my life will go on
as long as it goes on.
Sooner or later
other sorrow birds
will come my way.

As Astrid Lindgren said
in Mio My Mio:
The sorrow bird
always has something
he can sing about
doesn't he?

But later in a letter
Astrid Lindgren wrote:
You can't stop
the sorrow birds
from flying over your head
but you can stop them
from building a nest
in your hair.

With those wise words
it's time for me
to fly away.

# Thank You

This book is already extremely long, so in the interest of not adding more pages, I will list below all of the people who helped me, without naming the exact nature of that help. But no matter if they read the whole manuscript or found a single typo, every person below gave me support and encouragement in some way, and for that I am immensely grateful. My deepest apologies if there is anyone I have overlooked.

I do however want to thank Henry Chen for his beautiful artwork and cover layout. His elegant design captures both Sara's spirit and the essence of this book.

Warmest thanks to: Abbie Mitchell, Aileen Gao, Alexander Sugarman, Alli Liss, Anna von Friesen, Anneli Haake, Annika Nordqvist, Becky Vicars, Berlin Abraham, Beth Irikura, Britt St. John, Chris Coccoluto, Daniel Lind, David Chadwick, David Whitehead, Devon Fairchild, Ed Allnutt, Flora Sugarman, Harriet Barton, Jackie DeNieff, Jackie Pasqua, Joanna Huber, Johannes Vivers, Jose Alvarez, Julia Dillon, Khenpo Ugyen Tenzin, Lena Ahlström, Leon Clowes, Lisa Mercurio, Loraine Evans, Luise Mirow, Maggie Howard-Heretakis, Megan Glennon, Michelle Weintraub, Patricia Seminara, Sarah Bastos, Stockholm Poetry Society, Victoria Bastos Alvarez, Yrsa Keysendal och Flora Wiström of Skriv med Yrsa och Flora.

# Stay in Touch

Thank you so much for taking the time to read my book.

If you enjoyed what you read, please consider leaving a review on one of the many available platforms. Particularly Amazon, Goodreads, and BookBub.

If you need to reach me, my email address is florencewetzel@yahoo.com. You can also find me on Facebook as Florence Wetzel, and on Instagram as @florencewetzel108. I'm also on BookBub if you would like to follow me there.

If you would like to be informed of my new releases, just use this link to join my email list: https://florencewetzel.com/list

Printed in Great Britain
by Amazon

51287628R00212